Prostate Cancer

Sam S. Chang • Michael S. Cookson
Editors

Prostate Cancer

Clinical Case Scenarios

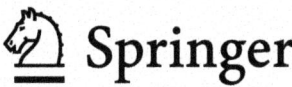

Editors
Sam S. Chang
Department of Urologic Surgery and
Oncology
Vanderbilt University Medical Center
Nashville, TN
USA

Michael S. Cookson
Department of Urology
University of Oklahoma Medical Center
Oklahoma City, OK
USA

ISBN 978-3-030-08755-5   ISBN 978-3-319-78646-9   (eBook)
https://doi.org/10.1007/978-3-319-78646-9

Printed on acid-free paper

This Springer imprint is published by the registered company Springer International Publishing AG
part of Springer Nature.
The registered company address is: Gewerbestrasse 11, 6330 Cham, Switzerland

Foreword

Willet Whitmore, often considered the father of urologic oncology and the first leader of the urology service at Memorial Sloan Kettering Cancer Center, was known for his visionary clinical care but also for his poignant witticisms. One of the latter was the comment that "There are more people making a living off of prostate cancer than there are dying from it." The statement was not meant to trivialize the suffering and death of too many patients with prostate cancer but to point out that legions of individuals were and still are involved in studying and treating the disease with little consensus among experts.

What also could be observed is that virtual libraries of literature exist on the clinical management of patients with prostate cancer. Do we really need another textbook on the topic? The indisputable answer is "yes." New data emerge; expert opinions shift, and novel treatment strategies develop. Published literature including dedicated texts is needed to chronicle and put in perspective these changes. Contemporary, state-of-the-art clinical care may be considered outdated or just plain wrong only a few years later.

Clinicians learn best by patient-centered discussion. This text is organized around defined clinical scenarios which are encountered routinely by physicians who care for patients with prostate cancer. The case-based format permits presentation of information of concise practical significance. The chapters run the gamut from screening controversies, utility of biomarkers, surveillance strategies, and innovative treatment. It manages to be comprehensive in 13 chapters by addressing the topics of most clinical relevance from detection of prostate cancer to management of patients with metastatic disease.

Mike Cookson and Sam Chang are superb editors for such a text. Both are widely recognized for their clinical acumen and surgical skills. They are leaders internationally in evaluating and treating patients with prostate cancer and are known for their dedication to patient care. Further, they have chosen a group of accomplished and well-recognized authors for each of the chapters. The clinical questions are sharply defined but the considerations which go in to addressing the questions are expansive. The authors help the reader understand the broad context and come to specific conclusions.

Patients put their very lives in the hands of physicians who provide their clinical care. In turn, it is an almost sacred responsibility for the clinician to remain informed and up to date, especially for a disease surrounded by so much controversy. If one were to put themselves into the position of a patient described in one of the 13 chapters, he would hope that his doctor had read this text.

Joseph A. Smith Jr.
Vanderbilt-Ingram Cancer Center
Nashville, TN, USA

Preface

The diagnosis, evaluation, and treatment of prostate cancer is continuously evolving. As editors, we are incredibly fortunate to have contributions by authors who are true leaders in the field. We have attempted to present clinical case scenarios that occur commonly yet do not have universally accepted single answers. The authors have succinctly presented data pertinent to these example patients and also present their thought processes as they decide how to proceed.

We are indebted to all of the authors for their contributions and want to recognize each and every one of our prostate cancer patients who live with this diagnosis and often times must determine their next step in an often times too confusing field.

Finally, our families provide encouragement, support, patience, and love—every single day—more than we can ever provide them.

Nashville, TN   Sam S. Chang
Oklahoma City, OK   Michael S. Cookson

Contents

Contributors

Marc A. Bjurlin, D.O. MSc. Department of Urology, NYU Langone Hospital—Brooklyn, Brooklyn, NY, USA

Matthew R. Cooperberg, M.D., M.P.H. Department of Urology, University of California, San Francisco, San Francisco, CA, USA

John Davis, M.D. Department of Urology, The University of Texas MD Anderson Cancer Center, Houston, TX, USA

Lucas W. Dean, M.D. Urology Service, Department of Surgery, Memorial Sloan Kettering Cancer Center, Sidney Kimmel Center for Prostate and Urologic Cancers, New York, NY, USA

Justin R. Gregg, M.D. Department of Urology, The University of Texas MD Anderson Cancer Center, Houston, TX, USA

William C. Jackson, M.D. Department of Radiation Oncology, University of Michigan, Ann Arbor, MI, USA

R. Jeffrey Karnes, M.D., F.A.C.S. Department of Urology, Mayo Clinic, Rochester, MN, USA

James T. Kearns, M.D. Department of Urology, University of Washington, Seattle, WA, USA

Aaron A. Laviana, M.D. Department of Urologic Surgery, Vanderbilt University Medical Center, Nashville, TN, USA

Daniel J. Lee, M.D. Department of Urology, Vanderbilt University Medical Center, Nashville, TN, USA

Daniel W. Lin, M.D. Department of Urology, University of Washington, Seattle, WA, USA

Division of Public Health Sciences, Fred Hutchinson Cancer Research Center, Seattle, WA, USA

William Lowrance, M.D., M.P.H. Division of Urology, Department of Surgery, Huntsman Cancer Institute, University of Utah, Salt Lake City, UT, USA

Christopher Martin, B.S. Division of Urology, Department of Surgery, Huntsman Cancer Institute, University of Utah, Salt Lake City, UT, USA

Todd M. Morgan, M.D. Department of Urology, University of Michigan, Ann Arbor, MI, USA

Bruno Nahar, M.D. Department of Urology, University of Miami Miller School of Medicine, Miami, FL, USA

Dipen J. Parekh, M.D. Department of Urology, University of Miami Miller School of Medicine, Miami, FL, USA

Daniel Parker, M.D. Department of Urology, University of Oklahoma Health Sciences Center, Oklahoma City, OK, USA

Benjamin H. Press Rutgers—New Jersey Medical School, Newark, NJ, USA

Chad Reichard, M.D. Department of Oncology, The University of Texas MD Anderson Cancer Center, Houston, TX, USA

Peter A. Reisz Department of Urologic Surgery, Vanderbilt University Medical Center, Nashville, TN, USA

Matthew J. Resnick, M.D., M.P.H., M.M.H.C. Department of Urologic Surgery, Vanderbilt University Medical Center, Nashville, TN, USA

Department of Health Policy, Vanderbilt University Medical Center, Nashville, TN, USA

Tennessee Valley VA Health Care System, Nashville, TN, USA

Cary N. Robertson, M.D., F.A.C.S. Division of Urology, Department of Surgery, Duke University Medical Center, Durham, NC, USA

Vidit Sharma, M.D. Department of Urology, Mayo Clinic, Rochester, MN, USA

Neal D. Shore, M.D., F.A.C.S. Carolina Urologic Research Center, Myrtle Beach, SC, USA

Matteo Soligo, M.D. Department of Urology, Mayo Clinic, Rochester, MN, USA

Daniel E. Spratt, M.D. Department of Radiation Oncology, University of Michigan, Ann Arbor, MI, USA

Kelly L. Stratton, M.D. Department of Urology, Stephenson Cancer Center, University of Oklahoma Health Sciences Center, Oklahoma City, OK, USA

Samir S. Taneja, M.D. Division of Urologic Oncology, Department of Urology, NYU Langone Health, New York, NY, USA

Karim A. Touijer, M.D. Urology Service, Department of Surgery, Memorial Sloan Kettering Cancer Center, Sidney Kimmel Center for Prostate and Urologic Cancers, New York, NY, USA

Vivek Venkatramani Department of Urology, University of Miami Miller School of Medicine, Miami, FL, USA

Samuel L. Washington III, M.D. Department of Urology, University of California, San Francisco, San Francisco, CA, USA

Chapter 1
Prostate Cancer Screening in African-American Men

Aaron A. Laviana, Peter A. Reisz, and Matthew J. Resnick

Clinical Case Scenario: A 44-year-old African-American Man with Two Brothers with Prostate Cancer Whose PSA Is 2.4.

Racial variation in prostate cancer incidence and outcomes has been well described. Men of African descent are disproportionately affected by this disease with an increased risk for cancer incidence, metastasis, and mortality [1–5]. The reasons for these disparities appear to be multifactorial and include variation in socioeconomic status, attitudes toward health care, and lifestyle factors including diet, access to care, and genetic predisposition [6–8]. Given this information, it would naturally follow that African-American men may stand to benefit from more aggressive screening for prostate cancer. This idea has been borne out by the literature, with several studies suggesting that more aggressive prostate-specific antigen (PSA) screening may begin to narrow observed disparities [9, 10].

In 2012, the United States Preventive Services Task Force (USPSTF) gave PSA screening a D recommendation for men of all ages. This recommendation was based primarily on the findings of two large randomized trials, the European Randomized Study of Screening for Prostate Cancer (ERSPC) and the Prostate, Lung, Colorectal, and Ovarian Cancer Screening Trial (PLCO), as well as evidence surrounding overdiagnosis and overtreatment resulting in potentially avoidable adverse side effects

A. A. Laviana, M.D. (✉) · P. A. Reisz
Department of Urologic Surgery, Vanderbilt University Medical Center, Nashville, TN, USA
e-mail: Aaron.a.laviana@vanderbilt.edu; peter.a.reisz@vanderbilt.edu

M. J. Resnick, M.D.
Department of Urologic Surgery, Vanderbilt University Medical Center, Nashville, TN, USA

Department of Health Policy, Vanderbilt University Medical Center, Nashville, TN, USA

Tennessee Valley VA Health Care System, Nashville, TN, USA
e-mail: matthew.resnick@vanderbilt.edu

© Springer International Publishing AG, part of Springer Nature 2018
S. S. Chang, M. S. Cookson (eds.), *Prostate Cancer*,
https://doi.org/10.1007/978-3-319-78646-9_1

in the context of small, predicted population-level benefits of opportunistic prostate cancer screening programs [11]. While the USPSTF recommendation addressed the increased risk of prostate cancer mortality in men of African origin, however, the panel stated that no firm conclusions could be extrapolated to this population given the relatively small numbers African-American men represented in the ERSPC and PLCO cohorts [12]. Following the most recent grade D recommendation, rates of PSA screening, prostate biopsy, and prostate cancer diagnosis decreased across all age groups in the United States [13]. Changes in the epidemiology of prostate cancer screening has fueled concerns that decreased prevalence of PSA screening will result in disease detection at more advanced stages, and that the potential reverse stage migration will preferentially impact African-American men [14].

Since 2012, longer-term follow-up of the ERSPC cohort has resulted in a more favorable yield of screening, reducing the number of men needed to be screened to prevent metastatic disease and death [15, 16]. There has also been an increased acceptance of active surveillance, thus reducing the burden of overtreatment and optimizing the balance of risk and benefit associated with prostate cancer detection and downstream treatment [17]. This recently resulted in a new draft USPSTF recommendation on PSA screening released for public commentary in 2017, which changed the recommendation for PSA screening in men ages 55–69 years from a "D" to a "C." The recommendation encourages "clinicians [to] inform men ages 55 to 69 years about the potential benefits and harms of PSA-based screening for prostate cancer" and encourage individualized decision-making about screening for prostate cancer after discussion with a clinician. This draft guideline also specifically addresses screening for prostate cancer in African-American men, as well as men with a family history of prostate cancer. Nevertheless, in both cases, the USPSTF again "is not able to make a separate, specific recommendation on PSA-based screening for prostate cancer" [18].

The clinical scenario of a "44-year-old African-American man with two brothers with prostate cancer whose PSA is 2.4" describes a man with two known factors that increase his risk for prostate cancer diagnosis and mortality, those being his African-American race and positive family history. The true extent to which these factors increase his risk for developing prostate cancer, however, is unclear. In this chapter, we systematically explore the literature in an effort to summarize our current understanding of these issues, in order to hopefully better counsel African-American men as we move forward.

Diagnosis and Screening

The drivers of observed prostate cancer racial disparities have been extensively investigated and describe the apparent contributions of both decreased access to care as well as the unique biology that characterizes the natural history of prostate cancer in African-American men. With higher prostate cancer incidence, more aggressive disease at diagnosis, higher rates of recurrence, metastatic disease, and increased mortality, more intensive screening protocols in this population are warranted [10, 19]. This opinion is supported by data from Powell et al. in 2014, who, using Surveillance, Epidemiology, and End Results (SEER) data, investigated the survival in African-American men during the pre-PSA testing era (1973–1994) compared to the current PSA testing era (1998–2005). The age-adjusted 5-year relative survival for prostate cancer was significantly lower for African-American men compared to European-American men during the pre-PSA era. This disparity narrowed, however, during the PSA era, suggesting that early detection in the high-risk African-American population is largely responsible for narrowing observed disparities in prostate cancer-specific survival [10]. Survival trends in men with metastatic prostate cancer included in SWOG trials also demonstrate overall improvement in survival for all men in the PSA-era with notable resolution of the disparity in survival between African-American men and European-American men. This improvement can be at least partially attributed to PSA screening [20]. The limitations in PSA screening have been well-detailed, and, along with more prudent PSA screening, a variety of risk stratification tools have been developed to improve patient selection for diagnostic biopsy.

Racial differences in PSA levels have been demonstrated in large, prospective, population-based cohorts. At baseline, the median PSA level in white men does not appear to differ from the median level observed in African-American men, but African-American men demonstrated a much more rapid increase in the PSA level over time after adjustment for prostate cancer and BPH medication use [21, 22]. African-American men without prostate cancer also have significantly higher PSA density when compared to Caucasian men [23]. Additionally, African-American men have been found to have higher serum PSA values at the time of prostate cancer diagnosis, correlating with increased tumor volume at the time of eventual radical prostatectomy [24]. Other studies examining prostate size, inflammation, and serum testosterone differences in African-American men did not demonstrate these factors to be contributory to higher observed PSA levels [25–27]. However, genetic variation in the PSA gene has been noted in African-American men compared to men of European descent and are thought to contribute to the difference in distribution of serum PSA between racial groups [28]. Certainly, these patterns in PSA level in men with and without prostate cancer must be taken into account when screening African-American men.

Epidemiologic and germline genetic analyses suggest that heredity plays a significant role in prostate cancer risk [29]. First-degree relatives of men with prostate cancer have twice the risk of developing prostate cancer as the general population [30]. This risk is increased in early-onset prostate cancer, with in excess of fourfold increased risk in men with first-degree relatives diagnosed before the age of 60 [31]. Twin studies also support this strong genetic familial contribution [32]. With the proliferation of DNA sequencing technology, there have been a multitude of efforts to identify the genetic loci associated with prostate cancer diagnosis and progression in both the germline and tumor genomes with the goal of improving both screening and treatment protocols. A number of genes and loci associated with the development of prostate cancer have been identified, with subsequent studies seeking to identify genomic markers unique to African-American men. The hereditary prostate cancer 1 susceptibility locus (HCP1) in ribonuclease L on chromosome 1q has been identified as a prostate cancer susceptibility gene, and variant alleles in this gene were demonstrated to be to be predictive of prostate cancer mortality in a population-based study [33]. The prevalence of this variant has been demonstrated to be significantly higher in African-American families than Caucasian families [34]. A single mutation in the HOXB13 gene has been found to be significantly more common in men with prostate cancer, especially in men with early-onset, familial prostate cancer [35]. This single mutation increases overall risk of prostate cancer fivefold [36]. BRCA1 and BRCA2 carriers have been demonstrated to be at increased risk for prostate cancer as well, especially for early-onset disease [37]. BRCA-associated cancers are also associated with more advanced, higher grade disease [38].

Genome-wide association studies (GWAS) have identified more than 100 prostate cancer risk alleles [36, 39]. No single genetic polymorphism or allele has demonstrated significant predictive value, but combinations of risk alleles have been studied as each allele added should incrementally increase the predictive value and potential clinical utility of these markers [40]. The vast majority of these studies have been performed in predominantly Caucasian cohorts with men of African descent representing a very small minority of patients. However, there have been several recent studies specifically seeking to characterize unique genetic polymorphisms in the African-American population [41–43]. Haiman et al. in 2011 performed a GWAS of prostate cancer in African-American men and identified a novel risk variant on chromosome 17q21 [44]. This is in addition to multiple independent risk variants at 8q24 [45]. These differences are summarized well by Faisal et al. in 2016 [46]. These authors also examined differences in androgen receptor (AR) mutations in African-American men, associating low AR signaling to anterior tumor location, which some studies have indicated is more prevalent in African-American men [47–49].

The AR is encoded on chromosome Xq11–12, and its transcriptional activity is inversely related to the number of CAG trinucleotide repeat sequences on its first exon [50]. Men with prostate cancer were more likely to have shorter CAG trinucleotide repeat sequences than men without the disease, and men with shorter CAG trinucleotide sequences were more likely to have advanced disease [51]. In a cohort of men without prostate cancer, African-American men were found to have significantly shorter CAG trinucleotide repeat sequences than white men [52]. However, subsequent studies have failed to demonstrate an association between AR CAG trinucleotide repeats and prostate cancer risk [53–55]. Expression of the androgen receptor itself is increased in radical prostatectomy specimens from African-American men when compared to Caucasian men [56]. The patterns of AR receptor pathway downstream activity are highly variable making racial comparisons difficult.

To this point, risk stratification based on genetic analysis has not been translated to meaningful changes in clinical protocols for screening Caucasian or African-American men. Nonetheless, efforts to optimize early detection of clinically significant disease and minimize overdetection have led to the development of commercial risk stratification instruments such as the Prostate Health Index (PHI), 4K Score, PCA3, ConfirmMDx™, SelectMDx™, Prolaris™, Oncotype Dx™, ProstaVision™, Promark™, and Decipher™, among others. Only PHI, 4 K Score™, PCA3™, and SelectMDx™ appear to currently have a role in screening. The extent to which these novel biomarkers stand to narrow observed racial disparities in prostate cancer outcomes remains largely unknown.

The Prostate Health Index (PHI) is calculated from serum measurements of PSA, free PSA, and pro2PSA and has been shown to predict clinically significant prostate cancer on biopsy with greater specificity than PSA alone [57, 58]. However, these studies have been performed with a predominance of Caucasian men. Recently, Schwen et al. evaluated the prognostic value of PHI in a cohort of 80 African-American men undergoing radical prostatectomy and demonstrated that a PHI >50 was associated with a fivefold increase in the odds of pT3 disease at the time of prostatectomy [59]. This data is similar to those of larger studies in men of European descent, supporting its clinical utility in African-American men in both screening and therapeutic management.

The 4-Kallikrein (4K™) score is calculated from serum measurements of total-PSA, free PSA, intact PSA, and human kallikrein-related peptidase 2. The 4K™ score has also demonstrated superior accuracy in predicting prostate cancer as well as high-grade disease when compared to PSA [60, 61]. The 4K™ score and PHI both have high diagnostic accuracy for prostate cancer with good sensitivity and specificity, and they are both able to predict high-grade disease [62]. However, the 4K™ score has not been specifically studied in an African-American population, so its utility in this unique population remains unknown.

Two other novel urinary biomarkers which merit discussion include SelectMDx™ and the Michigan Prostate Score (MiPS). SelectMDx™ measures mRNA levels of HOXC6 and DLX1 biomarkers in a post-digital rectal exam (DRE) urine sample [63]. The test improved the ability to predict clinically significant prostate cancer as well as avoid unnecessary biopsies. The Michigan Prostate Score combines urinary levels of PCA3 and TMPRSS2:ERG (T2ERG) combined with serum PSA. Urinary PCA3 and T2ERG have also been demonstrated to provide additional predictive value for identifying clinically significant prostate cancer in men of European descent. However, this notably did not hold true for African-American men [64]. Taken together, these data suggest that, while novel risk stratification tools may be useful, they may not be valid in the African-American population, and further studies characterizing performance in African-American populations are necessary.

In addition to novel biomarkers, magnetic resonance imaging of the prostate and MRI-fusion ultrasound-guided prostate biopsy have been shown to increase our ability to diagnose clinically significant cancer while decreasing the overdiagnosis of low-risk disease [65]. These tools have been validated in the African-American population for detecting clinically significant prostate cancer [66]. Several studies are ongoing to further evaluate the role of mpMRI in prostate cancer screening [67, 68]. However, these studies do not focus specifically on men of African origin and are European cohorts with relatively few men of African descent. Several studies suggest that African-American men are more likely to harbor anterior prostate tumors. These are more difficult to detect on digital rectal examination and more difficult to sample on prostate needle biopsy, potentially resulting in higher grade disease at the time of diagnosis and prostatectomy [47, 48]. However, a subsequent study by Kongnyuy et al. has not demonstrated a difference in the prevalence of anterior prostate lesions between African-American men and Caucasian men [69]. However, this study did demonstrate that African-American men with a prior negative transrectal ultrasound-guided prostate biopsy (TRUS Bx) and rising PSA are twice as likely to have an anterior prostate lesion, suggesting that African-American men may stand to benefit more from mpMRI to identify these lesions at risk for underdetection. Nevertheless, disparities in insurance coverage and treatment patterns have resulted in limited access to MRI screening and MRI-fusion biopsy [70] and make the use of mpMRI more complex in populations of lower socioeconomic status.

Evaluation

As described above, the natural history of prostate cancer in African-American men may be divergent from that of men of European descent, with African-American men presenting with higher grade disease and having less favorable oncological outcomes even after definitive local or locoregional treatment. Given this clinical scenario presented in the beginning, one should start with a thorough history and physical examination. This patient's history is notable for two brothers with prostate cancer. The age of onset is important, with more than a fourfold risk in individuals with first-degree relatives diagnosed before the age of 60 [31]. Direct questions should be asked regarding a family history of other malignancies as well, including breast, ovarian, and colorectal cancer, with the goal of identifying men potentially harboring BRCA2 or DNA repair gene mutations [71]. Evaluation of the patient's comorbid illnesses is essential, as this largely guides estimation of overall life expectancy which will undoubtedly influence critical management decisions. Physical examination must include a digital rectal examination for appropriate staging. Our patient's initial PSA is 2.4, but this must be evaluated in the context of his African-American race and strong family history of prostate cancer. His PSA should be checked again in several weeks to confirm this value, as there can be significant variation in PSA values from one measurement to another [72, 73].

The correct threshold PSA value to trigger biopsy remains controversial. Data from the Prostate Cancer Prevention Trial (PCPT) suggest that prostate cancer exists at all PSA levels and that a significant number of men with "normal" PSA levels harbor high-grade cancers [74]. The median serum PSA level for healthy men ages 30–49 years ranges between 0.6 and 0.78 ng/mL, and baseline PSA level was significantly higher for men aged 40–59 years who were diagnosed with prostate cancer versus those who were not [75]. African-American men demonstrate similar age-matched median PSA levels as compared to Caucasian men [20]. Per NCCN guidelines, clinicians should consider initial biopsy in men with a PSA of

2.6 or higher. The AUA does not recommend a PSA cutoff value. Notably, the European Urology Association (EUA) recommends earlier screening PSA in African-American men starting at 45 years old versus 50 years in Caucasian men. Kryvenko et al. in 2016 examined 414 radical prostatectomy specimens with Gleason 6 disease and found that African-American men had lower PSA values than white men, potentially suggesting that there should be a lower PSA threshold for biopsy in African-American men to achieve similar benefits associated with early detection [76].

Digital rectal examination is unable to assess reliably the anterior portion of the prostate gland, and thus anterior tumors may be missed. This is especially important in the African-American population, as some studies have noted a higher rate of anterior tumors in this population [47–49]. Faisal et al. also noted that anterior tumors are associated with lower PSA densities compared to posterior tumors [46]. Tumors in this location are more easily missed by DRE as well as prostate needle biopsy and, if they are truly more common in African-American men, may contribute to their presentation with higher grade disease, higher rates of progression, and worse oncologic outcomes [70]. The growing use of mpMRI and MRI-fusion prostate biopsy is expected to facilitate timely and accurate identification of anterior tumors. However, as mentioned above, there exist currently few data supporting the use of mpMRI in initial prostate cancer screening, nor is there evidence that mpMRI more accurately identifies anterior tumors. Thus, widespread adoption of MRI-based screening programs will likely be met with resistance owing to significant cost and unclear value.

In addition to prostate MRI, there are a multitude of biomarkers now available to supplement PSA and further guide the decision to proceed with prostate biopsy. As previous discussed, these biomarkers have generally not been validated in African-American populations. The decision to proceed with prostate biopsy must be individualized, weighting the predicted benefits associated with early prostate cancer detection against the potential harms of biopsy and downstream detection of potentially clinically insignificant disease. Certainly, a variety of prostate cancer screening nomograms may inform the potential benefits of biopsy.

The PCPT risk calculator was developed from analysis of the placebo cohort of the PCPT trial, which included 5519 men including the variables of PSA level, family history, digital rectal exam, prior negative biopsy, race, and age [77]. However, this cohort was 93% Caucasian, subsequently prompting validation of the PCPT calculator in a predominantly African-American population as represented by the Prostate Cancer Risk Assessment Program (PRAP) cohort at Fox Chase Cancer Center [78]. Of the 624 men included in this cohort, 382, or 61.2%, of the men were African-American, and the median PSA was 0.9% ng/mL. Altogether, the PCPT risk calculator accurately stratified prostate cancer risk in this young cohort with low baseline PSA level validating its use in this population. As a result, the use of this PCPT risk calculator, as well as others, may help to guide the conversation regarding prostate biopsy. Multivariate clinical risk prediction tools need to be further integrated into this decision-making process to maximize cancer detection, minimizing overdiagnosis, and offer patient-centered care plans. While the number of prostate cancer screening adjuncts is ever increasing, further investigation and validation of these tools in African-American populations must be completed before they become a part of our clinical lexicon.

Management

As stated previously, landmark studies with data as early as 1973 have found African-American men with prostate cancer to have worse disease-specific and overall survival rates than do their Caucasian counterparts [79]. African-American men not only tend to present with more advanced disease but also experience a survival disadvantage within stages [80]. Whether this is the result of genetic factors or health-care system, failure has been argued for decades but still remains to be determined [81]. For instance, some studies suggest a narrowing of the black-white survival gap with increasing age, which may be partially explained by differences in comorbidity. For example, in 1990, the mortality rate from heart disease among men aged 45–64 years was higher among African-Americans than whites (279 vs. 237 per 100,000, respectively); however, among men aged 65 and older, these mortality rate patterns were reversed (1375 vs. 1584 per 100,000, respectively) [82]. Therefore, it may be that fewer African-American men older than 65 years died from ischemic heart disease than otherwise might have been the case, given that those with more severe disease were removed through fatalities at younger ages. Resultantly, an improved overall survival among African-American men may reflect, in part, reduction in competing risks of mortality. Freeman et al. investigated this relationship further to characterize the effect of comorbidity at diagnosis on racial differences in survival among men with prostate cancer. This study found significant disparity in all-cause and prostate cancer-specific mortality between healthy Caucasian and African-American men. This disparity narrowed, however, as comorbidity increased. Resultantly, absence of a significant preexisting medical diagnosis was associated with a higher risk for excess mortality among African-American diagnosed with prostate cancer [83].

These racial differences were also pronounced in a SEER-Medicare study characterizing the relationship between prostate cancer recurrence and the risk of prostate cancer-specific mortality following definitive treatment among white, African-American, Hispanic, and Asian patients. In assessing patients from 1986 through 1998, the 75th percentile disease-free survival for black patients was 13 months less than for white patients (95% confidence interval [CI]: 6.2–19.8 months), 29.7 months less than that for Hispanic patients (95% CI: 4.4–55.0 months), and 39.1 months less than that for Asian patients (95% CI: 12.1–66.1 months) [83]. Furthermore, on multivariate analysis, African-American descent predicted earlier prostate cancer recurrence (shorter disease-free survival) among surgery patients. This earlier recurrence in African-American men may help explain their increased risk of prostate cancer mortality.

There is ample evidence that prostate cancer-specific outcomes among African-American men are inferior to their matched Caucasian counterparts. Despite these proposed differences in prostate cancer mortality and disease-free survival, access to care still remains a critical issue. In another SEER study evaluating whether having health insurance reduces racial disparities in the use of definitive therapy for high-risk prostate cancer, Mahal et al. found that African-American men were significantly less likely to receive definitive treatment after adjusting for sociodemographic characteristics and known disease-specific factors (adjusted odds ratio [AOR] = 0.60; 95% CI: 0.56–0.64, $p < 0.001$) [6]. There was a significant observed interaction between race and insurance status ($p = 0.01$) such that the adjusted odds ratio (AOR) for definitive treatment in African-American versus Caucasian men was markedly lower among uninsured (AOR 0.38, $p < 0.001$) versus insured men (AOR 0.62, $p < 0.001$) [84]. Ultimately, African-American men with high-risk prostate cancer were significantly less likely to receive potentially lifesaving definitive treatment when compared to white men, suggesting that expansion of health insurance coverage may help reduce racial disparities in the management of aggressive cancers.

Furthermore, with regard to access, African-American men were also found to be significantly less likely to receive treatment with curative intent than Caucasian man with no evidence that this disparity has narrowed with time. These differences appear more pronounced in high-risk than intermediate-risk disease, and after adjusting for treatment, demographics, and prognostic factors, African-American men had a higher risk of prostate cancer-specific mortality (adjusted hazard ratio, 1.12, 95% CI, 1.01–1.25, $p = 0.03$) [85]. Similar data by Zeliadt et al. found that the use of aggressive therapy has increased among Caucasian men over time but has declined among African-American men [86]. After controlling for age, grade, socioeconomic status, and comorbidity, African-American men were 26% less likely to receive aggressive therapy than Caucasian men (odds ratio 0.74, 95% confidence interval 0.70–0.79). Furthermore, despite evidence supporting the use of androgen deprivation therapy with external beam radiotherapy, the proportion receiving adjuvant ADT was 53.7% for Caucasian men and only 42.4% for African-American men ($p < 0.001$).

In order to characterize the effect of equal access to on racial disparities, Daskivich et al. sampled 1258 men with nonmetastatic prostate cancer at the Greater Los Angeles and Long Beach VA Medical Centers between 1998 and 2004 to assess whether an equal access health-care environment reduced barriers that influenced disparities in African-American men, including higher tumor risk at diagnosis, lower rates of surgical treatment, and less favorable cancer-specific survival [87]. Of note, the study revealed no significant differences in odds of higher tumor risk, Gleason score, or clinical stage for African-American versus Caucasian men. African-American men had similar odds of aggressive treatment as did Caucasians men for low-risk, intermediate-risk, and high-risk disease, suggesting that in the equal-access VA health-care setting, enhanced access may mitigate observed disparities in treatment intensity and outcomes.

Nevertheless, research by Cullen et al. also assessed a large racially diverse, longitudinal cohort with equal health-care access by examining men enrolled in the Center for Prostate Disease Research (CPDR) Multicenter National Database. Despite equal access to care, a greater odds of biochemical recurrence over time was observed for African-American versus Caucasian patients (HR = 1.28, CI = 1.11, 1.48, p = 0.0009) after adjustment for D'Amico risk stratum, comorbidity, pathological features, and PSA doubling time [88]. This has been also supported by Yamoah et al. who examined whether racial differences exist in the pattern of local disease progression among men treated with radical prostatectomy for localized prostate cancer. There were no observed differences in extraprostatic extension, positive surgical margins, lymph node involvement, or adverse pathologic features across race groups. However, among patients with > or = 1 adverse pathologic features, African-American men had higher rate of seminal vesicle invasion compared to Caucasian men (51% vs. 30%, p = 0.01) [89]. Upon adjusting for known predictors of adverse pathologic features, African-American race remained a predictor of seminal vesicle invasion, possibly reflecting racial differences in the biology of prostate cancer progression. This was further reinforced by a study by Faisal et al. who studied racial disparities in oncologic outcomes after radical prostatectomy through a median follow-up for 4.0 years [90]. When stratified by risk, African-American men with very low-, low-, or intermediate-risk prostate cancer who underwent radical prostatectomy were more likely to have adverse pathologic features including positive surgical margins and pathologic upgrading. Furthermore, African-American race was an independent predictor of biochemical recurrence among low-risk and intermediate-risk patients. In fact, biochemical-free survival for very low-risk African-American men was similar to low-risk Caucasian men and biochemical-free survival for low-risk African-American men was similar to that intermediate-risk white men.

Given the concern for unique and possible more aggressive pathologic features in African-American men, important concerns have been raised surrounding whether African-American men should be considered for active surveillance. The African-American population remains strongly underrepresented in the active surveillance literature, despite its potential for more aggressive pathology. Gökce et al. identified all studies reporting outcomes of the African-American population with low-risk prostate cancer than underwent active surveillance or treatment [91]. In 8 of 11 studies, African-American race was found to be associated with adverse pathological outcomes including positive surgical margins, upgrading, or upstaging. The other three studies reported no race-based difference in these parameters. African-American men were mainly found to have a higher rate of disease reclassification subsequent to active treatment. Given that African-American men with low-risk prostate cancer may have either a higher grade or volume of cancer not detected on routine evaluation, it is recommended that active surveillance in these men should be approached with caution. Unfortunately, existing favorable outcomes noted in largely Caucasian populations may not be applicable to African-American patients. Furthermore, these patients may best be served by an early confirmatory biopsy preceded by magnetic resonance imaging to optimally detect occult cancer

Fig. 1.1 Site of anterior and posterior dominant nodules. (**a**) In men at NCCN very low risk. (**b**) In men at upgraded NCCN very low risk. (Sundi, D., et al. Pathological examination of radical prostatectomy specimens in men with very low-risk disease at biopsy reveals distinct zonal distribution of cancer in black American men. J Urol 2013;191, 60–67, with permission)

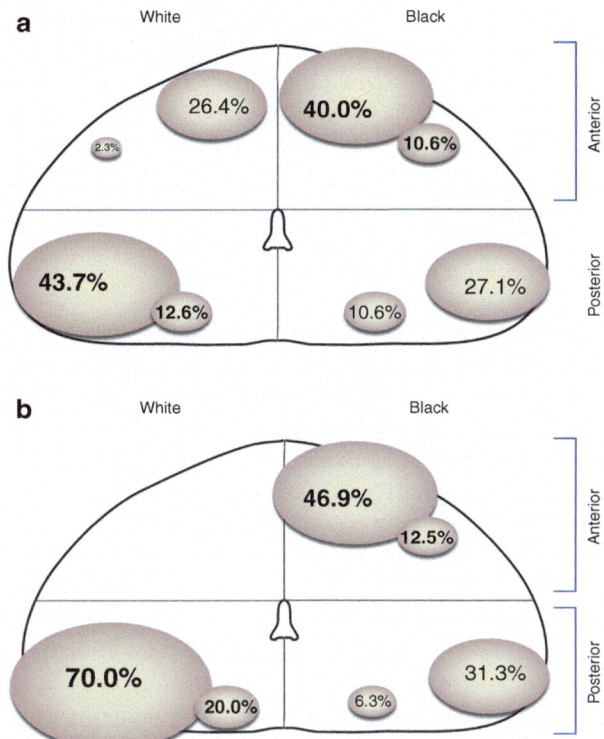

foci of higher-risk disease. Certainly, this is a critically important area of investigation that will inform clinical management in the future.

Though it has been postulated that African-American men may harbor more anterior prostate lesions that are undersampled by standard transrectal ultrasound-guided biopsy, potentially resulting in greater degree of Gleason score upgrading at radical prostatectomy, this remains debated [92]. Research by Sundi et al. assessed radical prostatectomy specimens in those with very low-risk prostate cancer [47]. They found that dominant nodules in black men were larger and more anterior (Fig. 1.1). Furthermore, in men who underwent pathological upgrading, the dominant nodule was also more frequently anterior in black than in white men. This argues that enhanced imaging or dedicated anterior zone sampling may improve detection these significant anterior tumors, potentially improving outcomes in black men considering active surveillance.

Despite it being well established that African-American men with prostate cancer exhibit more advanced disease at younger ages and are more likely to die of their disease compared to white men, data on how patient-reported changes in urinary, sexual, and bowel function vary after treatment remain sparse. Research by Tyson et al., utilizing data from the Comparative Effectiveness Analysis of Surgery and Radiation (CEASAR) study, assessed the association between race and patient-reported disease-specific function as measured using the 26-item Expanded Prostate

Table 1.1 Pretreatment function quartiles by race/ethnicity

White (n = 1835)	AA (n = 324)	Hispanic (n = 179)	p value	
Urinary irritative	88 (75–100)	88 (75–100)	81 (62–94)	0.013
Urinary incontinence	100 (85–100)	100 (73–100)	94 (68–100)	<0.001
Bowel function	100 (96–100)	100 (88–100)	100 (88–100)	0.003
Sexual function	75 (38–90)	67 (22–90)	65 (27–85)	<0.001

From Tyson MD, Alvarez J, Koyama T, et al. Racial variation in patient-reported outcomes following treatment for localized prostate cancer: results from the CEASAR Study. *European Urology.* 2017;72(2):307–14, with permission

Index Composite (EPIC) at baseline and 6 and 12 months after enrollment [93]. Importantly, African-American men reported a greater difference than Caucasian men with regard to urinary incontinence (adjusted difference-in-differences 8.4 points, 95% confidence interval 2.0–14.8; $p = 0.01$) (Table 1.1). No difference in bother scores was noted, and the overall proportion of explained variation attributable to race/ethnicity was relatively small with no clinically significant racial variation noted from the sexual, bowel, irritative voiding, or hormonal domains. Altogether, while these data demonstrate that incontinence at 1 year after radical prostatectomy may be worse among African-American compared to Caucasian men, the difference appears to be modest overall with treatment selection and baseline function explaining a much greater proportion of the variation in function after treatment. Nevertheless, these data are still critical in laying a foundation for ensuring high-quality decision-making among men of various racial and ethnic groups.

Furthermore, among African-American men receiving definitive therapy, radiation appears more common than surgery, and in those who undergo surgery, differences in surgical quality, oncological outcomes, and quality of life have emerged [94, 95]. From the available definitive treatment options for localized prostate cancer, more African-American men choose radiation over surgery [47, 93]. An evaluation of 66,836 men ≥65 years old with local or regional prostate cancer from 1986 to 1993 noted that African-American men were 70% as likely to undergo radical prostatectomy as Caucasian men. Sociodemographic and clinical characteristics could not fully account for this difference [96]. Even in the current era, after controlling for sociodemographic factors in the equal access Veterans Affairs System, African-American men continued to be less likely to pursue surgical therapy for prostate cancer management, though this difference was much less pronounced (23.2% vs. 25.9%) [97]. How observed differences in distribution of treatment map to outcome disparities, however, remains unknown.

Barocas et al. examined inpatient outcomes among 105,972 patients (13.2% African-American) undergoing radical prostatectomy from 1996 to 2007 in nonfederal hospitals [95]. In fully adjusted models, African-American men were less likely to use high-volume hospitals (OR 0.73, 95% CI 0.70–0.76; $p < 0.01$) and high-volume surgeons (OR 0.67, 95% CI 0.64–0.70; $p = <0.01$) than Caucasian men. Notably, high-volume hospitals and surgeons are two factors associated with higher-quality care. Comparing only those men undergoing surgery at high-volume hospitals with high-volume surgeons, African-American men still had higher odds of in-hospital mortality, transfusions, and a longer length of stay than Caucasian men. Older anthropomorphic data from as early as the nineteenth century has argued that narrow and deep pelvises [98] contribute to surgical complexity in African-American men. This is exacerbated by higher rates of obesity [99] and higher-volume disease [24].

African-American men are more likely to choose radiation therapy than surgical management than white men. In a cohort of 223 men (including 67 African-Americans) diagnosed with cancer on extended biopsy and counseled in a multidisciplinary clinic, African-American men were significantly more likely to choose radiation therapy for treatment than Caucasian men on multivariable analysis adjusted for age, PSA concentration, and prostate volume [100]. Among 102,486 men from the SEER database (17,594 of whom were African-Americans) with high-risk prostate cancer diagnosed between 2004 and 2010, African-American men were more likely to undergo radiation therapy (adjusted OR = 1.50; 95%CI: 1.44–1.57; $P < 0.001$) than Caucasian men [101].

Unfortunately, the uniformity of outcomes among races does not persist in the brachytherapy literature. In a study of 2268 men (including 270 African-Americans) receiving brachytherapy between 1990 and 2008 at Mount Sinai Medical Center, 30% of African-American men experienced biochemical failure at 10 years compared with only 16% of Caucasian men ($p = 0.002$) [102]. No differences in overall survival, cancer-specific survival, or metastasis-free survival were identified. In a study of 5360 men (339 of whom were African-American men) with clinical stage T1-3N0M0 prostate cancer who underwent brachytherapy between 1996 and 2006, African-American men had a significantly higher mortality rate (HR 1.77, 95% CI 1.3–2.5; $p < 0.001$) after adjusting for known prostate cancer risk factors, age, cardiovascular comorbidities, and income [103]. This study included only small percentage of African-American men and failed to fully adjust for comorbidities but still remains worrisome.

Multimodality therapy has proven benefit for men with locally advanced disease, but in a study of 3095 patients (including 326 African-American men) with cT3 or T4 disease by Lowrance et al., African-American men were less likely to receive multimodality therapy than Caucasian men (OR 0.67, CI 0.50–0.91; $P = 0.02$) [104]. Meanwhile, for men with metastatic prostate cancer, hormonal therapy remains the preferred treatment. Lu-Yao et al. investigated the records of 9110 men (1290 of whom were African-Americans) ≥65 years old that died of prostate cancer between 1991 and 2000. They found that 38% of African-American men and 25% of Caucasian men died of prostate cancer without receiving hormonal therapy (relative risk 0.83, 95% CI 0.79–0.86) [105].

Finally, at end of life, disparities in use of hospice care among men dying of prostate cancer have been identified. Bergman et al. evaluated 14,521 Medicare beneficiaries (1787 African-American men) who died of prostate cancer between 1992 and 2005 [106]. Approximately half of all men dying of prostate cancer in the cohort received hospice care, but African-American men were less likely than Caucasian men to receive hospice care (OR 0.78, 95% CI 0.68–0.88). With level 1 evidence that early palliative care leads to improvements in quality of life and mood as well as survival in oncologic patients [107], efforts to improve both access to palliative care and hospice care are critical to narrow observed racial disparities in high-value health-care utilization.

Conclusion

African-American men exhibit higher-risk prostate cancer and exhibit worse outcomes when compared to other racial and ethnic groups. There remain important knowledge gaps specifically surrounding the implications of this observed outcome disparity with respect to appropriateness and intensity of active surveillance in African-American men. Only approximately a tenth of the men in most active surveillance programs are African-American, yet the results are generalized as applying to all men equally. Nevertheless, because even "very low-risk" prostate cancer appears different pathologically and epidemiologically, African-American men must understand these risks when they electing management for prostate cancer. Most specifically, they must be aware that if they decide on active surveillance, aggressive cancer may be missed.

In the clinical scenario presented here, "a 44-year-old African American man with two brothers with prostate cancer whose PSA is 2.4" shared decision-making is of the utmost importance. Altogether, despite still being in an era where prostate MRI is still not approved for initial biopsy, we strongly feel the pendulum needs to be shifted to better take into consideration African-American men. Despite having a PSA of only 2.4, the patient's race and family history significantly increase his risk of harboring clinically significant, aggressive prostate cancer. To minimize the risk of a falsely negative prostate biopsy and with data supporting high rates of anterior lesions in African-American men, we support the use of performing a TRUS-fusion MRI guided biopsy to minimize the possibility of a false negative initial evaluation. Even if positive for only very low-risk prostate cancer, this information presented in this chapter suggests that we must be very cautious about placing this gentleman on active surveillance and would advocate for close monitoring with confirmatory biopsy and aggressive surveillance biopsy schedule. Even if this MRI-fusion TRUS biopsy is negative, these men should be followed more carefully with annual PSA's, with consideration of extending out the interval only if there is no change in value over several years. While we certainly do not minimize the burden of prostate cancer overtreatment, we need to better understand the natural history of the disease in African-American men before generalizing all prostate cancer recommendations to this unique subset of men at particular risk for adverse prostate cancer outcomes.

References

1. Howlader N, Noone AM, Krapcho M, Garshell J, Miller D, Altekruse SF, Kosary CL, Yu M. Ruhl J, Tatalovich Z, Mariotto A, Lewis DR, Chen HS, Feuer EJ, Cronin KA, editors. SEER Cancer Statistics Review, 1975–2011. Bethesda, MD: National Cancer Institute. http://seer.cancer.gov/csr/1975_2011/, based on November 2013 SEER data submission, posted to the SEER web site, April 2014.
2. Odedina FT, et al. Prostate cancer disparities in black men of African descent: a comparative literature review of prostate cancer burden among Black men in the United States, Caribbean, United Kingdom, and West Africa. Infect Agent Cancer. 2009;4:S2.

3. Sundi D, et al. African American men with very low-risk prostate cancer exhibit adverse onco-logic outcomes after radical prostatectomy: should active surveillance still be an option for them? J Clin Oncol. 2013;31:2991–7.
4. Resnick MJ, Canter DJ, Guzzo TJ, et al. Does race affect postoperative outcomes in patients with low-risk prostate cancer who undergo radical prostatectomy? Urology. 2009;73:620–3.
5. Powell IJ, Bock CH, Ruterbusch JJ, Sakr W. Evidence supports a faster growth rate and/or earlier transformation to clinically significant prostate cancer in black than in white American men, and influences racial progression and mortality disparity. J Urol. 2010;183:1792–6.
6. Mahal BA, et al. Getting back to equal: the influence of insurance status on racial disparities in the treatment of African American men with high-risk prostate cancer. Urol Oncol. 2014;32:1285–91.
7. Taksler GB, Keating NL, Cutler DM. Explaining racial differences in prostate cancer mortal-ity. Cancer. 2012;118:4280–9.
8. Cowen ME, Kattan MW, Miles BJ. A national survey of attitudes regarding participation in prostate carcinoma testing. Cancer. 1996;78:1952–7.
9. Evans S, et al. Clinical presentation and initial management of black men and white men with prostate cancer in the United Kingdom: the PROCESS cohort study. Br J Cancer. 2010;102:249–54.
10. Powell IJ, Vigneau FD, Bock CH, Ruterbusch J, Heilbrun LK. Reducing prostate cancer racial disparity: evidence for aggressive early prostate cancer PSA testing of African American men. Cancer Epidemiol Biomark Prev. 2014;23:1505–11.
11. Carlsson S, Vickers AJ, Roobol M, Eastham J, Scardino P, Lilja H, Hugosson J. Prostate cancer screening: facts, statistics, and interpretation in response to the US Preventive Service Task Force review. J Clin Oncol. 2012;30:2581–4.
12. Preventive Services Task Force US. Screening for prostate cancer: U.S. Preventive Services Task Force recommendation statement. Ann Intern Med. 2012;157(2):120–34.
13. Fleshner K, Carlsson SV, Roobol MJ. The effect of the USPSTF PSA screening recommenda-tion on prostate cancer incidence patterns in the USA. Nat Rev Urol. 2017;14:26–37.
14. Lee DJ, MAllin K, Graves A, Chang SS, et al. Recent changes in prostate cancer screening practices and epidemiology. J Urol. 2017;198(6):1230–40.
15. Buzzoni C, et al. Metastatic prostate cancer incidence and prostate-specific antigen testing: new insights from the European randomized study of screening for prostate cancer. Eur Urol. 2015;68:885–90.
16. Schroder FH, et al. The European randomized study of screening for prostate cancer—prostate cancer mortality at 13 years of follow-up. Lancet. 2014;382:2027–35.
17. Murphy DG, Loeb S. Prostate cancer: growth of AS in the USA signals reduction in overtreat-ment. Nat Rev Urol. 2015;12:604–5.
18. Bibbins-Domingo K, Grossman DC, Curry SJ. The US Preventive Service Task Force 2017 draft recommendation statement on screening for prostate cancer: an invitation to review and comment. JAMA. 2017;317:1949–50.
19. Shenoy D, et al. Do African-American men need separate prostate cancer screening guide-lines? BMC Urol. 2016;16:19.
20. Tangen CM, et al. Improved overall survival trends of men with newly diagnosed M1 prostate cancer: a SWOG phase III trial experience (S8494, S8894, & S9346). J Urol. 2012;188:1164–9.
21. Sarma AV, et al. Racial differences in longitudinal changes in serum prostate-specific antigen levels: the Olmsted County Study and the Flint Men's Health Study. J Urol. 2014;83:88–93.
22. McGreevy K, Rodgers K, Lipsitz S, Bissada N, Hoel D. Impact of race and baseline PSA on longitudinal PSA. Int J Cancer. 2006;118:1773–6.
23. Henderson RJ, Eastham JA, Culkin DJ, Kattan MW, Whatley T, Mata J, Venable D, Sartor O. Prostate-specific antigen (PSA) and PSA density: racial differences in men without prostate cancer. J Natl Cancer Inst. 1997;89:134–8.
24. Moul JW, et al. Prostate-specific antigen values at the time of prostate cancer diagnosis in African-American men. JAMA. 1995;274:1277–81.
25. Mavropoulos JC, et al. Do racial differences in prostate size explain higher serum prostate-specific antigen concentrations among black men? Urology. 2007;69:1138–42.

26. Zhang W, Sesterhenn IA, Connelly RR, Mostofi FK, Moul JW. Inflammatory infiltrate (prostatitis) in whole mounted radical prostatectomy specimens from black and white patients is not an etiology for racial difference in prostate specific antigen. J Urol. 2000;163:131–6.
27. Kubricht WS 3rd, Williams BJ, Whatley T, Pinckard P, Eastham JA. Serum testosterone levels in African-American and white men undergoing prostate biopsy. Urology. 1999;54:1035–8.
28. Bensen JT, et al. Genetic polymorphism and prostate cancer aggressiveness: a case-only study of 1,536 GWAS and candidate SNPs in African-Americans and European-Americans. Prostate. 2013;73:11–22.
29. Campbell MF, Wein AJ, Kavoussi LR, Partin AW, Peters CA, editors. Campbell-Walsh urology, Epidemiology, etiology, and prevention of prostate cancer. 11th ed. Philadelphia, PA: WB Saunders; 2016. p. 2546.
30. Goldgar DE, Easton DF, Cannon-Albright LA, Skolnick MH. Systematic population-based assessment of cancer risk in first-degree relatives of cancer probands. J Natl Cancer Inst. 1994;81:1600–8.
31. Lange EM. Male reproductive cancers: epidemiology, pathology, and genetics. In: Foulkes WD, Cooney KA, editors. . New York: Springer; 2010. p. 203–28.
32. Lichtenstein P, et al. Environmental and heritable factors in the causation of cancer—analyses of cohorts of twins from Sweden, Denmark, and Finland. N Engl J Med. 2000;343:78–85.
33. Lin DW, et al. Genetics variants in the LEPR, CRY1, RNASEL, IL4, and ARVCF genes are prognostic markers of prostate cancer-specific mortality. Cancer Epidemiol Biomark Prev. 2011;20:1928–36.
34. Cooney KA, et al. Prostate cancer susceptibility locus on chromosome 1q: a confirmatory study. J Natl Cancer Inst. 1997;89:955–9.
35. Ewing CM, et al. Germline mutations in HOVB13 and prostate-cancer risk. N Engl J Med. 2012;366:141–9.
36. Witte JS, et al. HOXB13 mutation and prostate cancer: studies of siblings and aggressive disease. Cancer Epidemiol Biomark Prev. 2013;22:675–80.
37. Eeles R, et al. The genetic epidemiology of prostate cancer and its clinical implications. Nat Rev Urol. 2014;11:18–31.
38. Castro E, et al. Germline BRCA mutations are associated with higher risk of nodal involvement, distant metastasis, and poor survival outcomes in prostate cancer. J Clin Oncol. 2013;31:1748–57.
39. Cooney KA. Inherited predisposition to prostate cancer: from gene discovery to clinical impact. Trans Am Clin Climatol Assoc. 2017;128:14–23.
40. Zheng SL, et al. Cumulative association of five genetic variants with prostate cancer. N Engl J Med. 2008;358:910.
41. Powell IJ, et al. Genes associated with prostate cancer are differentially expressed in African American and European American men. Cancer Epidemiol Biomark Prev. 2013;22:891–7.
42. Yamoah K, et al. Novel biomarker signature that may predict aggressive disease in African-American men with prostate cancer. J Clin Oncol. 2015;33:2789–96.
43. Tomlins SA, et al. Characterization of 1577 primary prostate cancers reveals novel biological and clinic opathologic insights into molecular subtypes. Eur Urol. 2015;68:555–67.
44. Haiman CA, et al. Genome-wide association study of prostate cancer in men of African ancestry identifies a susceptibility locus at 17q21. Nat Genet. 2011;43:570–3.
45. Freedman ML, et al. Admixture mapping identifies 8q24 as a prostate cancer risk locus in African-American men. Proc Natl Acad Sci U S A. 2006;103:14068–73.
46. Faisal FA, et al. Racial variations in prostate cancer molecular subtypes and androgen receptor signaling reflect anatomic tumor location. Eur Urol. 2016;70:14–7.
47. Sundi D, et al. Pathological examination of radical prostatectomy specimens in men with very low risk disease at biopsy reveals distinct zonal distribution of cancer in black American men. J Urol. 2014;191:60–7.
48. Tiguert R, Kabbani W, Sakr W, Gheiler EL, Pontes JE. Origin and racial distribution of glandular tissue in the anterior compartment of the prostate: an autopsy study. Prostate. 1999;39:310–5.

49. Pettaway CA, et al. Prostate specific antigen and pathological features of prostate cancer in black and white patients: a comparative study based on radical prostatectomy specimens. J Urol. 1998;160:437–42.
50. Beilin J, Ball EM, Favaloro JM, Zajac JD. Effect of the androgen receptor CAG repeat polymorphism on transcriptional activity: specificity in prostate and non-prostate cell lines. J Mol Endocrinol. 2000;25:85–96.
51. Giovannucci E, et al. The CAG repeat within the androgen receptor gene and its relationship to prostate cancer. Proc Natl Acad Sci U S A. 1997;94:3320–3.
52. Bennett CL, et al. Racial variation in CAG repeat lengths within the androgen receptor gene among prostate cancer patients of lower socioeconomic status. J Clin Oncol. 2002;20:3599–604.
53. Price DK, et al. Androgen receptor CAG repeat length and association with prostate cancer risk: results from the prostate cancer prevention trial. J Urol. 2010;184:2297–302.
54. Gilligan T, et al. Absence of a correlation of androgen receptor gene CAG repeat length and prostate cancer risk in an African-American population. Clin Prostate Cancer. 2004;3:98–103.
55. Freedman ML, et al. Systematic evaluation of genetic variation at the androgen receptor locus and risk of prostate cancer in a multiethnic cohort study. Am J Hum Genet. 2005;76:82–90.
56. Gaston KE, et al. Racial differences in androgen receptor protein expression in men with clinically localized prostate cancer. J Urol. 2003;170:990–3.
57. de la Calle C, Patil D, Wei JT, et al. Multicenter evaluation of the prostate health index to detect aggressive prostate cancer in biopsy naive men. J Urol. 2015;194:65–72.
58. Loeb S, Sanda MG, Broyles DL, et al. The prostate health index selectively identifies clinically significant prostate cancer. J Urol. 2015;193:1163–9.
59. Schwen ZR, Tosioan JJ, Sokoll LJ, et al. Prostate health index (PHI) predicts high-stage pathology in African American men. J Urol. 2016;90:136–40.
60. Vickers AJ, Gupta A, Savage CJ, et al. A panel of kallikrein marker predicts prostate cancer in a large, population-based cohort followed for 15 years without screening. Cancer Epidemiol Biomark Prev. 2011;20:255–61.
61. Nordstrom T, Vickers A, Assel M, Lilja H, Gronberg H, Eklund M. Comparison between the four-kallikrein panel and prostate health index for predicting prostate cancer. Eur Urol. 2015;68:139–44.
62. Russo GI, Regis F, Castelli T, et al. A systematic review and meta-analysis of the diagnostic accuracy of prostate health index and 4-Kallikrein panel score in predicting overall and high-grade prostate cancer. Clin genitour. Cancer. 2016;15:429–39.
63. Van Neste L, Hendriks RJ, Dijkstra S, et al. Detection of high-grade prostate cancer using a urinary molecular biomarker-based risk score. Eur Urol. 2016;70:740–8.
64. O'Malley PG, et al. Racial variation in the utility of urinary biomarkers PCA3 and T2ERG in a large multicenter study. J Urol. 2017;198:42–9.
65. Schoots IG, Roobol MJ, Nieboer D, et al. Magnetic resonance imaging-targeted biopsy may enhance the diagnostic accuracy of significant prostate cancer detection compared to standard transrectal ultrasound-guided biopsy: a systematic review and meta-analysis. Eur Urol. 2015;68:438–50.
66. Shin T, et al. Detection of prostate cancer using magnetic resonance imaging/ultrasonography image-fusion targeted biopsy in African-American men. BJU Int. 2017;120:233–8.
67. El-Shater Bosaily A, Parker C, Borwn LC, et al. PROMIS: prostate MR imaging study: a paired validating cohort study evaluating the role of multi-parametirc MRI in men with clinical suspicion of prostate cancer. Contemp Clin Trials. 2015;42:26–40.
68. Grenabo Bergdahl A, Wilderang U, Aus G, et al. Role of magnetic resonance imaging in prostate cancer screening: a pilot study within the Goteborg Randomised Screening Trial. Eur Urol. 2016;70:566–73.
69. Kongnyuy M, et al. The significance of anterior prostate lesions on multiparametric magnetic resonance imaging in African-American men. Urol Oncol. 2016;34:254.
70. Smith ZL, Eggener SE, Murphy AB. African-American prostate cancer disparities. Curr Urol Reports. 2017;18:81.

71. Carroll, PR, Parsons JK, Andriole, G, et al. NCCN Clinical Practice Guidelines Prostate Cancer Early Detection, Version 2.2017. www.nccn.org/professionals/physician_gls/pdf/prostate.pdf.
72. Eastham JA, Riedel E, Scardino PT, et al. Variation of serum prostate-specific antigen levels: an evaluation of year-to-year fluctuations. JAMA. 2003;289:2695–700.
73. Nordstrom T, Adolfsson J, Gronberg H, Eklund M. Repeat prostate-specific antigen tests before prostate biopsy decisions. J Natl Cancer Inst. 2016;108(12):djw165.
74. Thompson IM, Pauler DK, Goodman PJ, et al. Prevalence of prostate cancer among men with a prostate-specific antigen level ≤ 4.0 ng per milliliter. N Engl J Med. 2004;350:2239–46.
75. Loeb S, Roehl KA, Antenor JV, et al. Baseline prostate-specific antigen compared with median prostate-specific antigen for age group as predictor of prostate cancer risk in men younger than 60 years. Urology. 2006;67:316–20.
76. Kryvenko ON, Balise R, Soodana Prakash N, Epstein JI. African-American men with Gleason score 3+3=6 prostate cancer produce less prostate specific antigen than Caucasian men: a potential impact on active surveillance. J Urol. 2016;195:301–6.
77. Thompson IM, Ankerst DP, Chi C, et al. Assessing prostate cancer risk: results from the prostate cancer prevention trial. J Natl Cancer Inst. 2006;98:529–34.
78. Kaplan DJ, Boorjian SA, Ruth K, et al. Evaluation of the prostate cancer prevention trial risk calculator in a high-risk screening population. BJU Int. 2010;105:334–7.
79. Stanford JL, Stephenson RA, Coyle LM, et al. Prostate Cancer Trends 1973–1995. SEER Program. National Institutes of Health Publication 99-4543. Bethesda, MD: National Cancer Institute; 1999.
80. Merrill RM, Brawley OW. Prostate cancer incidence and mortality rates among whites and black men. Epidemiology. 1997;8:126–31.
81. Jepson C, Kessler LG, Portnoy B, Gibbs T. Black- white differences in cancer prevention knowledge and behavior. Am J Public Health. 1991;81:501–4.
82. National Center for Chronic Disease Prevention and Health Promotion. Chronic disease in minority populations. Atlanta, GA: Centers for Disease Control and Prevention; 1992.
83. Freeman VL, Durazo-Arvizu R, Keys L, et al. Racial differences in survival among men with prostate cancer and comorbidity at time of diagnosis. Am J Public Health. 2004;94(5):803–8.
84. Cohen JH, Schoenbach VJ, Kaufman JS, et al. Racial differences in clinical progression among Medicare recipients after treatment for localized prostate cancer (United States). Cancer Causes Control. 2006;17(6):803–11.
85. Mahal BA, Aizer AA, Ziehr DR, et al. Trends in disparate treatment of African-American men with localize prostate cancer across National Comprehensive Cancer Network risk groups. Urology. 2014;84(2):386–92.
86. Zeliadt SB, Potosky AL, Etzioni R, et al. Racial disparity in primary and adjuvant treatment for nonmetastatic prostate cancer: SEER-Medicare trends 1991 to 1999. Urology. 2004;64(6):1171–6.
87. Mahal BA, Ziehr DR, Aizer AA, et al. Getting back to equal: the influence of insurance status of racial disparities in the treatment of African American men with high-risk prostate cancer. Urol Oncol. 2014;32(8):1895–1.
88. Daskivich TJ, Kwan L, Dash A, Litwin MS. Racial parity in tumor burden, treatment choice and survival outcomes in men with prostate cancer in the VA healthcare system. Prostate Cancer Prostatic Dis. 2015;18:104–9.
89. Cullen J, Kuo H-C, Chen Y, et al. Prostate cancer outcomes for African American and Caucasian patients undergoing radical prostatectomy. JCO. 2017;35(6_suppl):40.
90. Yamoah K, Walker A, Spangler E, et al. African-American race is a predictor of seminal vesicle invasion following radical prostatectomy. Clin Genitourin Cancer. 2015;13(2):e65–72.
91. Faisal FA, Sundi D, Cooper JL, et al. Racial disparities in oncologic outcomes after radical prostatectomy: long-term follow-up. Urology. 2014;84(6):1434–41.
92. Gökce MI, Sundi D, Schaeffer E, Pettaway C. Is active surveillance a suitable option for African American men with prostate cancer? A systemic literature review. Prostate Cancer Prostatic Dis. 2017;20(2):127–36.

93. Tyson MD, Alvarez J, Koyama T, et al. Racial variation in patient-reported outcomes following treatment for localized prostate cancer: results from the CEASAR study. Eur Urol. 2017;72(2):307–14.
94. Sanchez-Ortiz RF, Troncoso P, Babaian RJ, et al. African-American men with nonpalpable prostate cancer exhibit greater tumor volume than matched white men. Cancer. 2006;107(1):75–82.
95. Barocas DA, Gray DT, Fowke JH. Racial variation in the quality of surgical care for prostate cancer. J Urol. 2012;188(4):1279–85.
96. Klabunde CN, Potosky AL, Harlan LC, Kramer BS. Trends and black/white differences in treatment for nonmetastatic prostate cancer. Med Care. 1998;36:1337–48.
97. Nambudiri VE, Landrum MB, McNeil BJ, et al. Understanding variation in primary prostate cancer treatment within the Veterans Health Administration. Urology. 2012;79:537–45.
98. Turner W. The index of the pelvic brim as a basis of classification. J Anat Physiol. 1885;20:125–43.
99. Ogden CL, Carroll MD, Kit BK, Flegal KM. Prevalence of childhood and adult obesity in the United States, 2011–2012. JAMA. 2014;311:806–14.
100. Swords K, Wallen EM, Pruthi RS. The impact of race on prostate cancer detection and choice of treatment in men undergoing a contemporary extended biopsy approach. Urol Oncol. 2010;28:280–4.
101. Ziehr DR, Mahal BA, Aizer AA, et al. Income inequality and treatment of African American men with high-risk prostate cancer. Urol Oncol. 2015;33:18.e7–18.e13.
102. Yamoah K, Beecham K, Hegarty SE, et al. Early results of prostate cancer radiation therapy: an analysis with emphasis on research strategies to improve treatment delivery and outcomes. BMC Cancer. 2013;13:23.
103. Winkfield KM, Chen MH, Dosoretz DE, et al. Race and survival following brachytherapy-based treatment for men with localized or locally advanced adenocarcinoma of the prostate. Int J Radiat Oncol Biol Phys. 2011;81(4):e345–50.
104. Lowrance WT, Elkin ED, Yee DS, et al. Locally advanced prostate cancer: a population-based study of treatment patterns. BJU Int. 2012;109:1309–14.
105. Lu-Yao G, Moore DF, Oleynick J, et al. Use of hormonal therapy in men with metastatic prostate cancer. J Urol. 2006;176:526–31.
106. Bergman J, Saigal CS, Lorenz KA, et al. Hospice use and high-intensity care in men dying of prostate cancer. Arch Intern Med. 2011;171(3):204–10.
107. Temel JS, Greer JA, Muzikansky A, et al. Early palliative care ofr patients with metastatic non-small-cell lung cancer. NEJM. 2010;363(8):733–42.

Chapter 2
Evaluation and Treatment for Older Men with Elevated PSA

Benjamin H. Press, Marc A. Bjurlin, and Samir S. Taneja

Clinical Case Scenario: A 76-year-old healthy man whose primary care physician orders a PSA that is 9 and wants to know what is his next best step.

The American Cancer Society estimates that in 2017, about 161, 350 new cases of prostate cancer will be diagnosed in the United States, accounting for 19% of new cancer diagnoses. They also estimate 26,730 prostate cancer-related deaths [1]. Prostate cancer is a disease of aging men, with an average age of diagnosis of 66 years. The probability of developing prostate cancer in men between 40 and 59 years of age is only 2.2% while 60% of cases are diagnosed in men over the age of 65 [1]. In a landmark study of autopsy results among men dying of causes of other than prostate cancer, occult prostate cancer detection was noted in 2%, 29%, 55%, and 64% in men in their 20s, 30s, 40s, 50s, and 60s, respectively [2]. More contemporary autopsy studies have estimated prostate cancer incidence of between 6–15%, 26%, 24–32%, 41–50%, 44–64%, and 59–86% in men in their 30s, 40s, 50s, 60s, 70s, and 80s [3, 4]. It is important to note that, in each of these age groups, elevated serum PSA level might suggest an even higher risk of prostate cancer.

B. H. Press
Rutgers—New Jersey Medical School, Newark, NJ, USA
e-mail: bhp36@njms.rutgers.edu

M. A. Bjurlin, D.O. MSc
Department of Urology, NYU Langone Hospital—Brooklyn, Brooklyn, NY, USA
e-mail: marc.bjurlin@nyumc.org

S. S. Taneja, M.D. (✉)
Division of Urologic Oncology, Department of Urology, NYU Langone Health, New York, NY, USA
e-mail: Samir.taneja@nyumc.org

© Springer International Publishing AG, part of Springer Nature 2018
S. S. Chang, M. S. Cookson (eds.), *Prostate Cancer*,
https://doi.org/10.1007/978-3-319-78646-9_2

Prostate cancer is largely an indolent malignancy, with diagnosis often preceding the risk of mortality by decades, resulting in a 5-year relative survival rate for all stages in the United States of >99% [1]. Five-year survival rates for local metastatic disease are also >99%; however, patients with distant metastatic disease have a 5-year survival rate of only 29%. A longitudinal trial in Sweden followed the progression of prostate cancer in 642 patients with a mean age of 72 years old for over 30 years [5–7]. At the 21-year follow-up, it was noted that the cause of death due to prostate cancer was inversely related to age. Among the age groups of <61, 61–70, 71–80, ≥81 years old, death due to prostate cancer decreased from 23%, 22%, 12%, to 4%, respectively, and the death due to other causes increased from 23%, 69%, 82%, to 96% [5]. These findings are similar to those found in a study by Albertson et al. which showed that, with increasing age, death due to prostate cancer and death due to other causes were inversely related, independent of Gleason score [8, 9].

The contemporary challenge for urologists evaluating men with elevated PSA levels, at risk of prostate cancer, is to balance the goal of early detection of potentially lethal prostate cancers, prior to metastasis or locoregional extension of disease, while avoiding the incidental over-detection of indolent disease. Given the increasing prevalence of prostate cancer with age, this challenge is magnified in the case of older men, in whom treatment is less likely to prolong longevity. A multifactorial approach should be taken when considering the approach to the older man with elevated PSA level. While the majority of such men would be at low risk of metastasis and prostate cancer death, occult high-grade disease does have the potential to cause morbidity, and even mortality, within the natural longevity of older men with few competing risks for mortality. As such, in the proposed case of the 76-year-old man who has an elevated PSA, a multifactorial approach should be considered when determining the necessity for biopsy or any other diagnostic step or even further follow-up. Evaluation of overall health and life expectancy, in combination of the use secondary tests can allow refined determination of risk and an individualized decision regarding the need for biopsy.

PSA Screening and USPSTF Recommendations

Prostate cancer mortality has substantially decreased over the past two decades. The prostate cancer death rate has been estimated to decrease 3% per year since 2009 [1]. A large amount of credit for this decrease in mortality can be attributed to the early detection of prostate cancer through community-based screening with prostate-specific antigen (PSA) [10–12]. Despite this, the United States Preventive Services Task Forces (USPSTF) issued a grade D recommendation against population-based PSA screening for men over the age of 75 in 2008, and then for all men in 2012 (Table 2.1), meaning, "there is moderate or high certainty that the service has no net benefit or that the harms outweigh the benefits"(https://www.

Table 2.1 Outline of USPSTF recommendations

Year	Population	Recommendation	Grade
2008	Men <75 years old	The USPSTF concludes that the current evidence is insufficient to assess the balance of benefits and harms of prostate cancer screening	I
2008	Men ≥75 years old	The USPSTF recommends against screening for prostate cancer	D
2012	Men	The USPSTF recommends against PSA-based screening for prostate cancer	D
Current (not final)	Men 55–69 years old	The USPSTF recommends that clinicians inform men ages 55 to 69 years about the potential benefits and harms of PSA–based screening for prostate cancer	C
	Men ≥70 years old	The USPSTF recommends against PSA-based screening for prostate cancer in men age 70 years and older	D

Adapted from https://www.uspreventiveservicestaskforce.org

uspreventiveservicestaskforce.org). In making the recommendations, the USPSTF members cited an inadequate magnitude of mortality reduction relative to the number of men treated, and a high rate of morbidity from treatment, resulting in reduction in quality of life.

The USPSTF recommendation was largely based on the conflicting results of two large studies [13]. The European Randomized Study of Prostate Cancer (ERSPC) randomized 162,243 men between the ages of 55 and 69 years between a receiving screening an average of every 4 years and not receiving screening. Their results demonstrated approximately a 20% reduction in prostate cancer mortality in those who underwent annual PSA screening [6, 14, 15]. Despite the mortality reduction observed, it was noted that treatment of 48 men was required to reduce one mortality. With increasing follow-up, this ratio has been shown to decline, illustrating the importance of prolonged survival to benefit from prostate cancer treatment. The Prostate, Lung, Colorectal, and Ovarian Cancer Screening Trial (PLCO) carried out in the United States randomized 76,693 patients between the ages of 55 and 74 years to either annual screening with PSA and digital rectal exam or "usual care," which could in fact include screening [16]. This trial found no difference in prostate cancer mortality between those who received annual screening and those receiving usual care [17, 18]. The PLCO outcomes have been subsequently questioned given the extremely high rate of contamination in the control arm, with nearly as many men receiving PSA testing as the screened arm [19]. Despite the consensus that the PLCO trial outcomes are largely meaningless in assessing the impact of screening, the USPSTF has utilized the trial as a basic premise of their recommendations. The USPSTF guidelines differ from the recommendations of the American Urological Association (AUA) and the European Association of Urology (EAU), which both recommend PSA screening based on life expectancy [20, 21]. Since their 2012 recommendation, the USPSTF has revised their guidelines on PSA screening for men between the ages of 55 and 69. They advise physicians to have individualized discussion of screening with patients in this age group. However, they still advise against PSA-based screening for men aged 70 and older (https://screeningforprostatecancer.org/).

Impact of USPSTF Recommendations

The USPSTF statement on PSA-based screening for prostate cancer has had a significant impact on current urologic practice. Aslani et al. report that at University Hospitals Case Medical Center in Ohio, PSA-based screening has significantly decreased among all age groups after March 2009 after an upward trend for the previous year. They reported the most significant decrease was in the age group of 50–59 years [22]. Similarly, a study from the Veterans Affairs demonstrated that PSA testing decreased in the age groups of 40–54 years, 55–74 years, and ≥75 years by 3%, 2.7%, and 2.2%, respectively, following the publication of the PLCO and ERSPC. In an analysis of male Medicare beneficiaries, Ross et al. reported that PSA-based screening declined among men aged 75 years and older by 1.6% [23]. Comparing 2010 and 2013 results from the National Health Interview Survey, Drazer et al. confirmed that screening rates significantly declined in men between ages 50 to 59 years from 33.2% to 24.8%, ages 60 to 74 years from 51.2% to 43.6%, and ages 75 years or older from 43.9% to 37.1% [24].

Overdiagnosis and Overtreatment

The utility of PSA-based screening is limited by the fact that PSA is not a cancer-specific marker. In fact, many nonneoplastic conditions such as benign prostatic hyperplasia (BPH), urinary tract infection (UTI), and prostatitis can lead to an elevated PSA in men [25]. The debate over screening for prostate cancer rooted in what often follows an abnormally elevated PSA in clinical practice [5]. Over one million men undergo transrectal ultrasound-guided biopsy every year in Europe and the United States. Indications for biopsy include abnormal digital rectal exam (DRE) and/or an elevated PSA. A PSA level > 4 ng/mL leading to a prostate biopsy is common in clinical practice. Although often a safe and well-tolerated procedure, it is not without a risk of complications, including sepsis, hematuria, rectal bleeding, hematospermia urinary tract infections, and urinary retention [26]. Hospitalization following biopsy, while rare, has been reported in 0.6–4.1% of patients [27].

While the morbidity and cost of biopsy are a major concern, the detection of indolent disease can have major consequences for the patient. Predictions of overdiagnosis of indolent prostate cancer have been estimated to be as low as 1.7% and as high as 67% [28]. Detection of indolent and clinically insignificant can lead to unnecessary treatment, future biopsies on surveillance, and increased patient anxiety related to the cancer diagnosis. From a practical standpoint, the diagnosis of cancer can make it difficult for patient's to secure life insurance, health benefits, and employment in rare instances. The most important thing urologists can learn from the population-based screening trials and the randomized comparisons of treatment and surveillance is the necessity for prolonged longevity in order for men to benefit from treatment. Careful assessment of competing risks for mortality is an essential first consideration before biopsy rather than before treatment.

The need for this assessment is highlighted in the results of two large-scale clinical trials comparing observation vs. intervention: the Prostate Testing for Cancer and Treatment (ProtecT) and the Prostate Cancer Intervention versus Observation Trial (PIVOT). The results of the ProtecT trial revealed that both all-cause and prostate cancer-specific mortality were not significantly different between patients under active monitoring, patients who underwent surgery, and patients who were treated with radiation. However, there was a significant increase in metastases and disease progression in men who did not undergo treatment with curative intent [29]. While the initial reports of ProtecT study suggest that treatment, in general, would have little benefit among men with longevity of 10 years or more, the results must be viewed with caution. As the trial was a randomization following detection, the majority of men in both treatment and observation arms harbored low-risk cancers with likely long lead times to cancer mortality. When considering men with higher risk cancers alone, or more advanced stage at presentation, the benefits of therapy are not well defined by the study. One would expect that treatment of cancers with shorter lead time to treatment would offer greater benefit.

The results of the PIVOT trial revealed similar results, but the trial has been greatly criticized for several reasons. The investigators reported that there was a nonsignificant difference in all-cause mortality between patients on observation and patients who underwent radical prostatectomy. There was an increase in disease progression and additional treatment in patients on observation vs. patients who underwent surgery [30]. It was noted in the first report of the study, published in 2012, that the inclusion criteria of the trial were expanded to include older men, and men with greater comorbidity, due to poor accrual by the original, intended criteria. As a result, men in this study most often died of competing risks long before prostate cancer would have harmed them. In an updated 20-year follow-up report, at a median follow-up of 12.7 years, the PIVOT study continued to demonstrate no improvement in survival among men treated [31]. At 19.5 years of follow-up, 65% of enrolled men were dead, with 20, 40, and 50% dead at 5, 10, and 12 years, respectively. Less than 10% of men died of prostate cancer, but two thirds died overall [31]. The high early death rate leaves too few men alive at prolonged follow-up to demonstrate benefit for treatment, despite longer lead time. Despite its shortcomings, the PIVOT trial clearly demonstrates the importance of carefully selecting men for prostate cancer evaluation who have adequate anticipated longevity to benefit from prostate cancer treatment.

Life Expectancy Tools

Determining the life expectancy of the patient is essential in making decisions regarding curative treatment of prostate cancer. The NCCN stresses the use of life expectancy in evaluating patients with prostate cancer, stating: "Life expectancy estimation is critical to informed decision-making in prostate cancer early detection and treatment" [32]. The NCCN recommends using the Social Security Administration tables or the World Health Organization's life tables [32].

Prior studies have evaluated the ability of clinicians to predict life expectancy in patients with prostate cancer [33]. Considering the NCCN Guidelines recommending curative treatment if life expectancy is ≥10 years [32], Koch et al. evaluated the ability of physicians to predict life expectancy compared with actuarial tables in 261 patients who underwent radical prostatectomy. The authors estimated that their physician assessment of life expectancy was in agreement with the actuarial estimations [34]. These results are similar with the accuracy reported by Krahn et al. who reported that 191 urologists were able to predict life expectancy of less than 10 years for 18 patient scenarios at an 82% accuracy rate when compared to a Markov model incorporating age and comorbidity [35]. Incorporating actual patient data, Walz et al. examined the accuracy of 19 clinicians in predicting 10-year survival of 50 patients undergoing definitive treatment for prostate cancer. Analysis using area under the curve (AUC) for receiver operating characteristic (ROC) curves found that attending urologists had a predictive ability of 0.67 (0.60–0.72), residents 0.69 (0.64–0.74), and medical students 0.67 (0.58–0.76) [36]. The lack of experience influencing predictive ability was echoed by the results of Leung et al. that found that sex, level of training, type of healthcare institution, and medical specialty had no impact on the ability to predict life expectancy [37]. Thus, although formal tools provide quick measures, a careful evaluation of a patient's health and comorbidities may be adequate to predict life expectancy.

Assessment of Cancer Risk

Longevity assessment must be contemplated within the context of cancer aggressiveness. Men with aggressive malignancies may benefit from diagnosis and treatment regardless of a shortened longevity, particularly if presenting at an advanced stage. In the case of prostate cancer, lead time from diagnosis to symptoms is heavily influenced by Gleason score and tumor stage. Initial assessment should include a discussion of local symptoms including obstructive/irritative lower tract symptoms, pain, and hematuria. Exam should include a careful digital rectal inspection of the gland contour, margins, and consistency. Suspicion of locally advanced disease, or local disease of sufficient volume to create symptoms, should prompt biopsy and further evaluation.

In most cases, men do not present with obvious evidence of locally advanced disease or local symptoms, and as such, additional tests may be useful in further risk stratification prior to consideration of biopsy.

Alternatives to PSA-Based Screening: Biomarkers

While no biomarker, to date, carries sufficient accuracy to determine the presence of clinically significant, or potentially lethal, prostate cancer, several PSA derivatives, secondary urine and blood biomarkers, and imaging techniques have been evaluated for their ability to refine risk assessment in men with elevated PSA.

PSA Derivatives

Due to the limitations of PSA, attempts have been made to improve it as a diagnostic tool. These attempts include stratifying PSA by age [38], PSA velocity [39, 40], the ratio of PSA to the prostate volume (PSAD) [41], and isoforms of PSA [42]. Among these tools, PSA velocity and PSAD are the tools most frequently used in clinical practice. PSA velocity has been shown to be significantly associated with high-risk cancer [43]. However, it requires multiple measurements and stringent follow-up for truly accurate measurements. PSAD has been shown to be a predictive marker for disease progression [44, 45]. One of the limitations to PSAD is that it requires an ultrasound in order to properly determine prostate volume, [46] and accuracy of ultrasound is operator dependent. It has been documented that PSA is correlated with age and prostate volume [38]. Current literature is inconsistent on the utility of the use of age-stratified PSA ranges for biopsy indication, with some studies advocating for its use [47, 48] and other studies advocating to maintain the status quo [49, 50].

Free PSA

PSA exists as both a bound and unbound form. Men with prostate cancer have a lower percentage of the unbound form (%fPSA) than men without prostate cancer [51, 52]. The use of %fPSA has been approved by the US Food and Drug Administration (FDA) for men with PSA between 4 and 10 ng/mL. In a multicenter study of 773 men with PSA between 4 and 10 ng/mL, Catalona et al. found that using a 25% fPSA cutoff detected 95% of prostate cancer and avoided 20% of unnecessary biopsies [53]. Ankerst et al. showed that %fPSA was an earlier indicator of prostate cancer. Using thresholds of 25% and 15% fPSA, fPSA detected prostate cancer earlier than PSA in 71 and 34% of cases, respectively [54].

Prostate Health Index

Prostate Health Index (phi) combines PSA, fPSA, and (−2)proPSA, an isoform of fPSA. The PDA has approved phi for men with PSA levels between 4 and 10 ng/mL. In a multicenter prospective trial, Loeb et al. revealed that, for men over 50 with PSA between 4 and 10 ng/mL, phi was a superior predictor of prostate cancer than each of the individual components of the index [55]. At a cutoff of 28.6 for phi, 30.1% of patients with either benign or clinically insignificant prostate cancer could have been spared an unnecessary biopsy, compared to only 21.7% of patients using %fPSA alone [51]. In a multicenter study with two independent prospective cohorts, it was found that phi had a higher specificity for prostate cancer than PSA and %fPSA at 95% sensitivity. The authors also found that at a phi cutoff of 24, 41% and 36% of unnecessary biopsies were avoided in the two cohorts [56].

4Kscore

The 4Kscore is a panel of kallikrein markers (tPSA, fPSA, intact PSA, human kallikrein 2) combined with age, DRE, and prior prostate biopsy results to predict the probability of high-grade prostate cancer on biopsy. While it is not FDA approved, the 4Kscore is certified by the Clinical Laboratory Improvement Amendments (CLIA) program of the Centers for Medicare and Medicaid Services. 4Kscore was validated in a prospective study in the United States of 1012 patients across 26 centers. They found that for detection of Gleason ≥ 7, 4Kscore demonstrated superior predictive ability when compared to a modified PCPTRC (AUC 0.82 vs. 0.74). A cutoff of $4K \geq 9\%$ was shown to avoid 43% of biopsies while only missing 2.4% of high-grade disease [57]. In another validation study, Vickers et al. found that the addition of the kallikrein panel improved high-grade cancer detection compared with a model based on PSA, age, and DRE (AUC 0.78 vs. 0.70) and a model based on PSA and age (AUC 0.76 vs. 0.64). In this study, using a $4K \geq 20\%$ cutoff, the number of biopsies would reduce by over 50% while missing 12% of high-grade disease [58]. The ability of 4Kscore to predict detection of high-grade prostate cancer on biopsy has been further established in a number of studies [59–62]. 4Kscore has also been shown to be significantly associated with [63] and improved prediction [64] of higher pathologic grade in radical prostatectomy specimens.

Prostate Cancer Antigen 3

Prostate cancer antigen 3 (PCA3) is a noncoding mRNA that is overexpressed in prostatic tumors compared to nonneoplastic prostate tissue [65, 66]. It is detectable in urine after digital rectal exam. The FDA has approved the use of PCA3 with a cutoff of 25 in men older the age of 50 with at least one prior negative biopsy. The National Comprehensive Cancer Network (NCCN) recommends a PCA3 cutoff of 35 in patients with PSA >3 ng/mL with previous negative biopsy when considering a repeat biopsy [67]. Published studies have shown superiority of PCA3 of predicting outcomes of prostate biopsy when compared to PSA [68] and %fPSA [69]. Despite this, evidence points to PCA3 as a supplementary tool, rather than a sole predictor of prostate cancer. In a multicenter trial of 859 men, Wei et al. demonstrated that while using a PCA3 cutoff of 20 would avoid a repeat biopsy in 46% of patients. However, this cutoff fails to diagnose prostate cancer in 12% of patients and high-grade cancer in 3% of patients. When applying the same cutoff to the initial biopsy, a diagnosis of aggressive cancer is missed in 13% of patients [70].

Predictive Nomograms

A number of attempts have been made to develop predictive models for predicting prostate cancer. One of these models includes the Prostate Cancer Prevention Trial (PCPT) Risk Calculator. This model was developed from the placebo arm of the PCPT [71] and uses PSA, DRE, family history, previous biopsy status, age, and race to predict biopsy results. The risk calculator was modified in 2012 to incorporate a prediction of high vs. low-grade prostate cancer [72]. An additional nomogram was generated from the ERSPC [73] that utilizes a series of calculators to determine risk of prostate cancer, including a differentiation between low and high-grade disease (http://www.prostatecancer-riskcalculator.com/). These two nomograms have been compared to one another with inconsistent results. Studies have demonstrated the superiority of ERSPC [74], the superiority of PCPT [75], and no significant difference between the two [76].

Nomograms have also been developed to predict recurrence of disease following radical prostatectomy [77, 78]. The preoperative nomogram prior to radical prostatectomy incorporates PSA, clinical stage, and Gleason score on prostate biopsy [77]. The postoperative nomogram includes PSA, Gleason score, extracapsular extension, surgical margin, seminal vesicle invasion, and lymph node invasion [78]. Validated nomograms for predicting recurrence following radiation therapy [79, 80] and predicting metastases following radiation therapy have also been developed [81].

Prostate MRI

Prostate magnetic resonance imaging (MRI) is becoming increasingly used in clinical practice in the diagnostic pathway for prostate cancer [82]. MRI may add value as both a pre-biopsy risk assessment tool that may influence the decision whether to perform biopsy as well as a noninvasive method for tumor localization to direct targeted biopsy [83]. Prostate MRI along with the MRI suspicion score (Prostate Imaging Reporting and Data System [PI-RADS]) has demonstrated the potential for improved individualized risk stratification. For example, several studies have shown an association between the level of suspicion on pre-biopsy MRI and outcomes of biopsy [84–86]. In particular, MRI suspicion score has consistently served as a strong predictor of the likelihood of significant prostate cancer on subsequent biopsy, even in the context of other clinical risk factors [87–89]. Our institutional experience has demonstrated that clinically significant cancer ($\geq$Gleason score 7) is found on MRI-targeted biopsy of PI-RADS 2, 3, 4, and 5 lesions in 5%, 14%, 49%, and 82%, respectively [90]. Other studies have shown results in-line with our experience [91]. PI-RADS v2 scores have also been shown to be predictive of cancer aggressiveness on radical prostatectomy [92]. A recent pooled data meta-analysis assessing the performance of prostate MRI in prostate cancer detection reported a specificity of 88% and sensitivity of 74%, with a negative predictive value of 65% to 94% [93].

Quantitative metrics of diffusion-weighted MRI, such as apparent diffusion coefficient (ADC), correlate well with disease aggressiveness [94]. ADC has been shown to predict Gleason score [95], risk of adverse surgical pathology [96, 97], progression on active surveillance [94, 96, 98], and biochemical relapse after surgery [99–101]. Despite the strong correlation of ADC with Gleason score, the confidence intervals for low, intermediate, and high risk are widely overlapping [102], making it impossible to predict Gleason score solely on the basis of diffusion weighted imaging alone.

Nomograms and risk calculators have been developed to help identify patients at risk for prostate cancer prior to biopsy, allowing counseling on both cancer risk and need for biopsy. Historically, nomogram variables have included PSA, percentage of free PSA, digital rectal examination, and prostate volume, but recently nomograms have been enhanced through incorporation of MRI findings to predict both overall and clinically significant cancer risk [103–105]. When applying our institutional nomograms to the study index patient (76-year-old biopsy-naïve man with a PSA of 9 ng/mL), we see that if he underwent a MRI and was found to have a PI-RADS 2 lesion with a prostate volume of 65 grams, his estimated risk of clinically significant cancer (≥Gleason score 7) is about 30%, and perhaps he may avoid a biopsy (Fig. 2.1) [105]. Alternatively, if he was found to have a PI-RADS 5 lesion, his risk of clinically significant cancer increases to >95%. These predictive nomo-

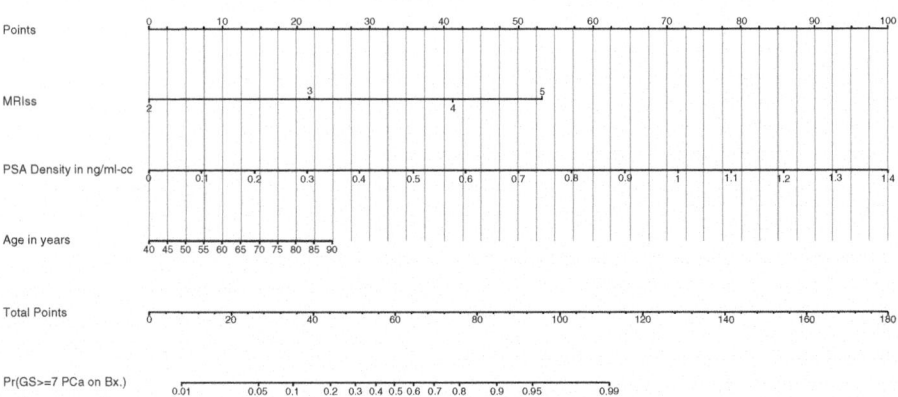

Fig. 2.1 Nomogram prediction model for predicting overall Gleason ≥7 prostate cancer in men without a prior biopsy. (Adapted from: Bjurlin MA SS et al. Prediction of Prostate Cancer Risk Among Men Undergoing Combined MRI-Targeted and Systematic Biopsy using Novel Pre-Biopsy Nomograms that Incorporate MRI findings. Urology. 2017 Nov 16. pii: S0090–4295(17)31185–8, with permission)

grams may potentially reduce unnecessary prostate biopsies and overdiagnosis while improving risk stratification counseling.

In addition to the ability to aid in prediction of clinically significant cancer, MRI can provide valuable information regarding disease volume, local advancement, and risk of subsequent symptoms. In older patients with marginally elevated serum PSA levels, this information can help in determining the necessity or urgency for biopsy.

Special Considerations in Elderly Patients

A different approach must be taken when dealing with prostate cancer in elderly patients when compared to younger patients. In contrast to their younger counterparts, a more thorough investigation into an elderly patient's cognitive function, social situation, financial status, and life expectancy to ensure the benefits of screening and treatment outweigh potential harm to the patient. The International Society of Geriatric Oncology (SIOG) assembled a group to review screening tools for elderly cancer patients, and they found that a full geriatric assessment (GA) was still superior to the screening tools [106]. The GA is a multidisciplinary approach to diagnosis and treatment of elderly patient that includes demographic, social, nutritional, and cognitive status [107]. Some studies have reported that GA is predictive of mortality and other adverse events of treatment [108, 109]. One of the limitations of this assessment is that it is very time-consuming, and not all patients will actually require such a thorough investigation [33].

The SIOG recommends that the health status of an elderly patient be evaluated with a G8 and mini-Cog™. If indicated, these screening measures should be followed by a simplified GA and then a comprehensive GA if necessary [110]. The SIOG task force found that the G8 was the most robust in screening for patients who require further evaluation with a comprehensive GA [33, 111]. While the Mini-Mental State Examination (MMSE) remains the clinical standard for detecting cognitive function in elderly patients, like the comprehensive GA, it is time-consuming [112] and is under copyright protection [113]. The mini-Cog™ has been shown to be a comparable diagnostic tool as the MMSE [106, 114].

An Optimized Diagnostic Approach

In approaching the elderly patient with elevated PSA, it is critical to communicate the goals of evaluation to the patient. Knowing that the prevalence of occult prostate cancer is quite high on the basis of age alone, the simple diagnosis of any cancer is not an ideal goal for patient or physician. Instead, an optimized biopsy approach should allow for the detection of potentially lethal prostate cancer, while minimizing the detection of indolent cancer and biopsy utilization in general. Such an optimized approach is further individualized through careful longevity assessment,

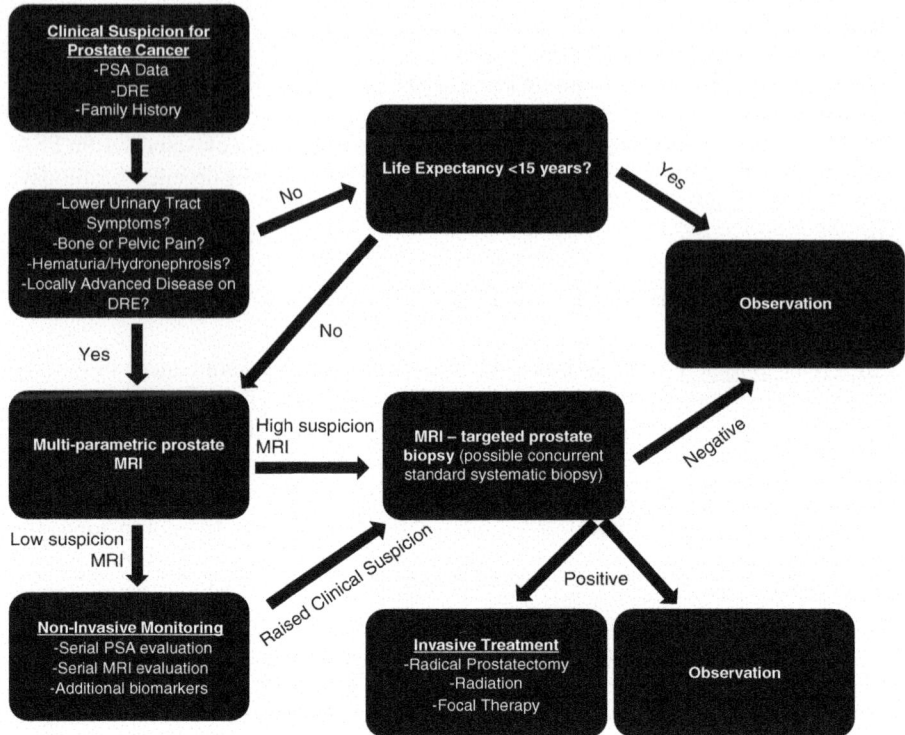

Fig. 2.2 Potential diagnostic algorithm for men >75 years of age presenting with elevated PSA

history and physical exam, and selective use of secondary testing to refine risk assessment (Fig. 2.2).

In men presenting with clinical symptoms of prostate cancer, locally advanced disease, or rapidly rising serum PSA (suggestive of high-grade disease), biopsy should be performed in order to rule out high-grade prostate cancer. In the locally advanced, symptomatic patient, treatment is often indicated, regardless of age.

In our patient, a presumably asymptomatic, healthy 76-year-old man with no immediate competing risks for mortality, the decision for biopsy can be difficult. Despite apparent good longevity, the majority of men in this age group will not benefit from aggressive biopsy and treatment, with regard to either improved survival or avoidance of local symptoms. In our practice, we have advocated an approach of image-based risk stratification using prostate MRI. In this case, MRI could be used to help with the decision for biopsy, through assessment of suspicion score and local tumor burden, and could be used to direct biopsy to the most suspicious regions of the prostate, if indicated. Given the desire to avoid indolent cancer detection, limited sampling, through MRI-directed cores alone, may be a reasonable consideration in patients with intermediate to high suspicion MRI abnormalities, in order to rule out aggressive cancer.

In men with equivocal or low suspicion MRI findings, biopsy could be deferred in view of the unclear benefit of therapy in men of this age group. We have previously demonstrated cancer detection rates segregated by MRI suspicion scores among men without previous biopsy (Table 2.2) [115]. In our experience, suspicion scores of 2 and 3 are rarely associated with high-grade cancer, while a high probability of high-grade disease is associated with suspicion scores 4 and 5 (Fig. 2.3). Among men with low MRI suspicion scores, if continued suspicion is noted on the basis of rising PSA over time, markedly elevated PSA, or strong genetic risk, additional risk stratification through nomograms or secondary biomarkers could be contemplated.

Many have suggested the use of secondary biomarkers such as 4Kscore, phi, or PCA3 to allow for the selection of men who might benefit from prostate MRI prior to biopsy selection. We have previously demonstrated that use of the PCA3 biomarker to select men for prostate MRI would result in reduction of biopsies by 76.4% but would miss 47.5% of occult high-grade disease [116]. Alternatively, use of the MRI to segregate men at high risk (suspicion scores 4 and 5) and low risk (suspicion scores 2 and 3), biopsy of men at high risk, and PCA3 selection of men

Table 2.2 Cancer detection rates by MRI suspicion score

MRI suspicion score	Cancer detection rate (% of patients)		
	Gleason ≥7	Gleason 6	Negative
4 or 5	69.1	16.8	14.1
2 or 3	12.4	21.5	66.1

Adapted from Mendhiratta N, Rosenkrantz AB, Meng X, Wysock JS, Fenstermaker M, Huang R et al. Magnetic Resonance Imaging-Ultrasound Fusion Targeted Prostate Biopsy in a Consecutive Cohort of Men with No Previous Biopsy: Reduction of Over Detection through Improved Risk Stratification. J Urol. 2015;194(6):1601–6, with permission

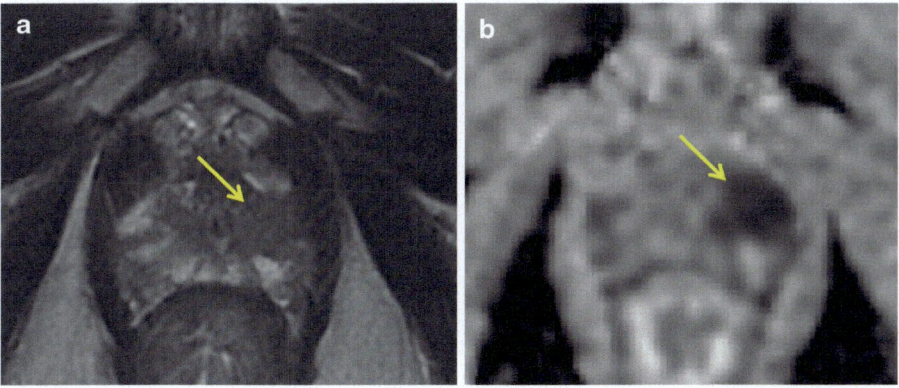

Fig. 2.3 Case of a 76-year-old man with a PSA of 9.4 and normal DRE. Imaging demonstrated a PI-RADS 5 region of suspicion in the left anterior apex (yellow arrows) on (**a**) T2-weighted MRI and (**b**) diffusion weighted MRI, apparent diffusion coefficient (ADC) map. MRI-ultrasound fusion targeted biopsy revealed Gleason 8 (4 + 4) and Gleason 9 (4 + 5) prostate cancer

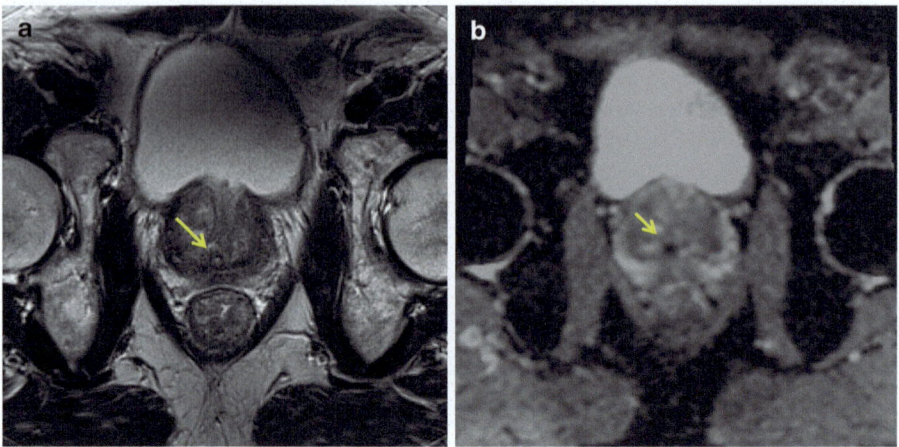

Fig. 2.4 Case of a 72-year-old man with a PSA of 4.6 and a normal DRE. Imaging demonstrated a PI-RADS 2 region of suspicion in the midline base (yellow arrows) on (**a**) T2-weighted MRI sequence and (**b**) diffusion-weighted MRI, apparent diffusion coefficient (ADC) map. As the patient and physician were hesitant to proceed to biopsy, a 4Kscore was measured to be 17%, placing him at intermediate risk for the detection of high-grade cancer. On this basis, MRI-ultrasound fusion targeted biopsy was performed revealing high-grade prostatic intraepithelial neoplasia in the targeted sample and no cancer on systematic biopsy

in need of biopsy would allow reduction of biopsy utilization by 36.3% but would only miss 4.9% of high-grade cancers. On this basis, we have utilized a strategy of biomarker-based risk stratification among men with equivocal indications for biopsy and low-risk prostate MRI (Fig. 2.4).

Ultimately, the decision to defer biopsy in this population is not necessarily a permanent one. As decisions for care remain dynamic, a period of deferral may allow better assessment of PSA velocity, patient health and stability, and may allow the patient time to research and contemplate the risks and benefits of biopsy and potential cancer detection. Use of prostate MRI for risk stratification allows selection of a group of men in whom deferral of biopsy would seem to have little risk.

Conclusions

The management of elderly men presenting with asymptomatic, elevated PSA levels requires careful consideration of the risks and benefits or biopsy, cancer detection, and subsequent cancer treatment. In men over the age of 75 years, presenting with elevated PSA levels, the prevalence of prostate cancer is high, but the benefit of treatment is not clear. The risk of prostate cancer mortality declines as men age and competing risks of mortality grow. As such, careful consideration of patient health and longevity is the mainstay of decision-making in this clinical scenario. If healthy, further evaluation with prostate MRI, predictive nomograms, and/or selective biomarkers may allow selection of men at greatest risk harboring cancers which potentially affect natural longevity. In this manner, not all men presenting at age 76 with modestly elevated PSA will require biopsy, but those few who remain at risk of prostate cancer mortality might still benefit from early detection.

References

1. Cancer Facts and Figures. 2017. https://www.cancer.org/content/dam/cancer-org/research/cancer-facts-and-statistics/annual-cancer-facts-and-figures/2017/cancer-facts-and-figures-2017.pdf.
2. Sakr WA, Grignon D, Crissman J, Heilbrun L, Cassin B, Pontes JJE, et al. High grade prostatic intraepithelial neoplasia (HGPIN) and prostatic adenocarcinoma between ages of 20–69: autopsy study of 249 cases. In Vivo. 1993;8:439–43.
3. Soos G, Tsakiris I, Szanto J, Turzo C, Haas PG, Dezso B. The prevalence of prostate carcinoma and its precursor in Hungary: an autopsy study. Eur Urol 2005;48(5):739-44.
4. Zlotta AR, Egawa S, Pushkar D, Govorov A, Kimura T, Kido M, et al. Prevalence of prostate cancer on autopsy: cross-sectional study on unscreened Caucasian and Asian men. J Natl Cancer Inst. 2013;105(14):1050–8.
5. Johansson JE, Andren O, Andersson SO, Dickman PW, Holmberg L, Magnuson A, et al. Natural history of early, localized prostate cancer. JAMA. 2004;291(22):2713–9.
6. Johansson JE, Holmberg L, Johansson S, Bergstrom R, Adami HO. Fifteen-year survival in prostate cancer. A prospective, population-based study in Sweden. JAMA. 1997;277(6):467–71.
7. Popiolek M, Rider JR, Andren O, Andersson SO, Holmberg L, Adami HO, et al. Natural history of early, localized prostate cancer: a final report from three decades of follow-up. Eur Urol. 2013;63(3):428–35.
8. Albertsen PC, Hanley JA, Fine J. 20-year outcomes following conservative management of clinically localized prostate cancer. JAMA. 2005;293(17):2095–101.
9. Albertsen PC, Hanley JA, Gleason DF, Barry MJ. Competing risk analysis of men aged 55 to 74 years at diagnosis managed conservatively for clinically localized prostate cancer. JAMA. 1998;280(11):975–80.
10. Hugosson J, Carlsson S, Aus G, Bergdahl S, Khatami A, Lodding P, et al. Mortality results from the Goteborg randomised population-based prostate-cancer screening trial. Lancet Oncol. 2010;11(8):725–32.
11. Klotz L. Prostate cancer overdiagnosis and overtreatment. Curr Opin Endocrinol Diabetes Obes. 2013;20(3):204–9.
12. Schroder FH, Hugosson J, Roobol MJ, Tammela TL, Ciatto S, Nelen V, et al. Screening and prostate-cancer mortality in a randomized European study. N Engl J Med. 2009;360(13):1320–8.
13. Chou R, Croswell JM, Dana T, Bougatsos C, Blazina I, Fu R, et al. Screening for prostate cancer: a review of the evidence for the U.S. Preventive Services Task Force. Ann Intern Med. 2011;155(11):762–71.
14. Schroder FH, Hugosson J, Roobol MJ, Tammela TL, Ciatto S, Nelen V, et al. Prostate-cancer mortality at 11 years of follow-up. N Engl J Med. 2012;366(11):981–90.
15. Schroder FH, Hugosson J, Roobol MJ, Tammela TLJ, Zappa M, Nelen V, et al. Screening and prostate cancer mortality: results of the European randomised study of screening for prostate cancer (ERSPC) at 13 years of follow-up. Lancet. 2014;384(9959):2027–35.
16. Andriole GL, Crawford ED, Grubb RL 3rd, Buys SS, Chia D, Church TR, et al. Mortality results from a randomized prostate-cancer screening trial. N Engl J Med. 2009;360(13):1310–9.
17. Andriole GL, Crawford ED, Grubb RL 3rd, Buys SS, Chia D, Church TR, et al. Prostate cancer screening in the randomized prostate, lung, colorectal, and ovarian cancer screening trial: mortality results after 13 years of follow-up. J Natl Cancer Inst. 2012;104(2):125–32.

18. Pinsky PF, Parnes HL, Andriole G. Mortality and complications after prostate biopsy in the prostate, lung, colorectal and ovarian cancer screening (PLCO) trial. BJU Int. 2014;113(2):254–9.
19. Shoag JE, Mittal S, Hu JC. Reevaluating PSA testing rates in the PLCO trial. N Engl J Med. 2016;374(18):1795–6.
20. Carter HB, Albertsen PC, Barry MJ, Etzioni R, Freedland SJ, Greene KL, et al. Early detection of prostate cancer: AUA guideline. J Urol. 2013;190(2):419–26.
21. Mottet N, Bellmunt J, Bolla M, Briers E, Cumberbatch MG, De Santis M, et al. EAU-ESTRO-SIOG guidelines on prostate cancer. Part 1: screening, diagnosis, and local treatment with curative intent. Eur Urol. 2017;71(4):618–29.
22. Aslani A, Minnillo BJ, Johnson B, Cherullo EE, Ponsky LE, Abouassaly R. The impact of recent screening recommendations on prostate cancer screening in a large health care system. J Urol. 2014;191(6):1737–42.
23. Ross JS, Wang R, Long JB, Gross CP, Ma X. Impact of the 2008 US Preventive Services Task Force recommendation to discontinue prostate cancer screening among male Medicare beneficiaries. Arch Intern Med. 2012;172(20):1601–3.
24. Drazer MW, Huo D, Eggener SE. National Prostate Cancer Screening Rates after the 2012 US preventive services task force recommendation discouraging prostate-specific antigen-based screening. J Clin Oncol. 2015;33(22):2416–23.
25. Morote Robles J, Ruibal Morell A, Palou Redorta J, de Torres Mateos JA, Soler Rosello A. Clinical behavior of prostatic specific antigen and prostatic acid phosphatase: a comparative study. Eur Urol. 1988;14(5):360–6.
26. Loeb S, Vellekoop A, Ahmed HU, Catto J, Emberton M, Nam R, et al. Systematic review of complications of prostate biopsy. Eur Urol. 2013;64(6):876–92.
27. Bjurlin MA, Wysock JS, Taneja SS. Optimization of prostate biopsy: review of technique and complications. Urol Clin North Am. 2014;41(2):299–313.
28. Loeb S, Bjurlin MA, Nicholson J, Tammela TL, Penson DF, Carter HB, et al. Overdiagnosis and overtreatment of prostate cancer. Eur Urol. 2014;65(6):1046–55.
29. Hamdy FC, Donovan JL, Lane JA, Mason M, Metcalfe C, Holding P, et al. 10-year outcomes after monitoring, surgery, or radiotherapy for localized prostate cancer. N Engl J Med. 2016;375(15):1415–24.
30. Wilt TJ, Brawer MK, Jones KM, Barry MJ, Aronson WJ, Fox S, et al. Radical prostatectomy versus observation for localized prostate cancer. N Engl J Med. 2012;367(3):203–13.
31. Wilt TJ, Jones KM, Barry MJ, Andriole GL, Culkin D, Wheeler T, et al. Follow-up of prostatectomy versus observation for early prostate cancer. N Engl J Med. 2017;377(2):132–42.
32. NCCN Guidelines Version 3.2016.
33. Sammon JD, Abdollah F, D'Amico A, Gettman M, Haese A, Suardi N, et al. Predicting life expectancy in men diagnosed with prostate cancer. Eur Urol. 2015;68(5):756–65.
34. Koch MO, Miller DA, Butler R, Lebos L, Collings D, Smith JA. Are we selecting the right patients for treatment of localized prostate cancer? Results of an actuarial analysis. Urology. 1998;51(2):197–202.
35. Krahn MD, Bremner KE, Asaria J, Alibhai SM, Nam R, Tomlinson G, et al. The ten-year rule revisited: accuracy of clinicians' estimates of life expectancy in patients with localized prostate cancer. Urology. 2002;60(2):258–63.
36. Walz J, Gallina A, Perrotte P, Jeldres C, Trinh QD, Hutterer GC, et al. Clinicians are poor raters of life-expectancy before radical prostatectomy or definitive radiotherapy for localized prostate cancer. BJU Int. 2007;100(6):1254–8.
37. Leung KM, Hopman WM, Kawakami J. Challenging the 10-year rule: the accuracy of patient life expectancy predictions by physicians in relation to prostate cancer management. Can Urol Assoc J. 2012;6(5):367–73.
38. Oesterling JE, Jacobsen SJ, Chute CG, Guess HA, Girman CJ, Panser LA, et al. Serum prostate-specific antigen in a community-based population of healthy men. Establishment of age-specific reference ranges. JAMA. 1993;270(7):860–4.

39. Carter HB, Pearson JD, Metter J, Brant LJ, Chan DW, Andres R, et al. Longitudinal evaluation of prostate-specific antigen levels in men with and without prostate disease. JAMA. 1992;267(16):2215–20.
40. Loughlin KR. PSA velocity: a systematic review of clinical applications. Urol Oncol. 2014;32(8):1116–25.
41. Verma A, St Onge J, Dhillon K, Chorneyko A. PSA density improves prediction of prostate cancer. Can J Urol. 2014;21(3):7312–21.
42. Guazzoni G, Nava L, Lazzeri M, Scattoni V, Lughezzani G, Maccagnano C, et al. Prostate-specific antigen (PSA) isoform p2PSA significantly improves the prediction of prostate cancer at initial extended prostate biopsies in patients with total PSA between 2.0 and 10 ng/ml: results of a prospective study in a clinical setting. Eur Urol. 2011;60(2):214–22.
43. Loeb S, Kettermann A, Ferrucci L, Landis P, Metter EJ, Carter HB. PSA doubling time versus PSA velocity to predict high-risk prostate cancer: data from the Baltimore Longitudinal Study of Aging. Eur Urol. 2008;54(5):1073–80.
44. Barayan GA, Brimo F, Begin LR, Hanley JA, Liu Z, Kassouf W, et al. Factors influencing disease progression of prostate cancer under active surveillance: a McGill University Health Center cohort. BJU Int. 2014;114(6b):E99–E104.
45. San Francisco IF, Werner L, Regan MM, Garnick MB, Bubley G, DeWolf WC. Risk stratification and validation of prostate specific antigen density as independent predictor of progression in men with low risk prostate cancer during active surveillance. J Urol. 2011;185(2):471–6.
46. Loeb S, Han M, Roehl KA, Antenor JA, Catalona WJ. Accuracy of prostate weight estimation by digital rectal examination versus transrectal ultrasonography. J Urol. 2005;173(1):63–5.
47. Oesterling JE, Jacobsen SJ, Cooner WH. The use of age-specific reference ranges for serum prostate specific antigen in men 60 years old or older. J Urol. 1995;153(4):1160–3.
48. Partin AW, Criley SR, Subong EN, Zincke H, Walsh PC, Oesterling JE. Standard versus age-specific prostate specific antigen reference ranges among men with clinically localized prostate cancer: a pathological analysis. J Urol. 1996;155(4):1336–9.
49. Borer JG, Sherman J, Solomon MC, Plawker MW, Macchia RJ. Age specific prostate specific antigen reference ranges: population specific. J Urol. 1998;159(2):444–8.
50. Crawford ED, Leewansangtong S, Goktas S, Holthaus K, Baier M. Efficiency of prostate-specific antigen and digital rectal examination in screening, using 4.0 ng/ml and age-specific reference range as a cutoff for abnormal values. Prostate. 1999;38(4):296–302.
51. Partin AW, Brawer MK, Subong EN, Kelley CA, Cox JL, Bruzek DJ, et al. Prospective evaluation of percent free-PSA and complexed-PSA for early detection of prostate cancer. Prostate Cancer Prostatic Dis. 1998;1(4):197–203.
52. Christensson A, Björk T, Nilsson O, Dahlén U, Matikainen M-T, Cockett ATK, et al. Serum prostate specific antigen complexed to α 1-Antichymotrypsin as an indicator of prostate cancer. J Urol. 1993;150(1):100–5.
53. Catalona WJ, Partin AW, Slawin KM, Brawer MK, Flanigan RC, Patel A, et al. Use of the percentage of free prostate-specific antigen to enhance differentiation of prostate cancer from benign prostatic disease—a prospective multicenter clinical trial. JAMA. 1998;279(19):1542–7.
54. Ankerst DP, Gelfond J, Goros M, Herrera J, Strobl A, Thompson IM Jr, et al. Serial percent free prostate specific antigen in combination with prostate specific antigen for population based early detection of prostate cancer. J Urol. 2016;196(2):355–60.
55. Loeb S, Sanda MG, Broyles DL, Shin SS, Bangma CH, Wei JT, et al. The prostate health index selectively identifies clinically significant prostate cancer. J Urol. 2015;193(4):1163–9.
56. de la Calle C, Patil D, Wei JT, Scherr DS, Sokoll L, Chan DW, et al. Multicenter evaluation of the prostate health index to detect aggressive prostate cancer in biopsy naive men. J Urol. 2015;194(1):65–72.
57. Parekh DJ, Punnen S, Sjoberg DD, Asroff SW, Bailen JL, Cochran JS, et al. A multi-institutional prospective trial in the USA confirms that the 4Kscore accurately identifies men with high-grade prostate cancer. Eur Urol. 2015;68(3):464–70.

58. Vickers A, Cronin A, Roobol M, Savage C, Peltola M, Pettersson K, et al. Reducing unnecessary biopsy during prostate cancer screening using a four-kallikrein panel: an independent replication. J Clin Oncol. 2010;28(15):2493–8.
59. Braun K, Sjoberg DD, Vickers AJ, Lilja H, Bjartell AS. A four-kallikrein panel predicts high-grade cancer on biopsy: independent validation in a community cohort. Eur Urol. 2016;69(3):505–11.
60. Bryant RJ, Sjoberg DD, Vickers AJ, Robinson MC, Kumar R, Marsden L, et al. Predicting high-grade cancer at ten-core prostate biopsy using four kallikrein markers measured in blood in the ProtecT study. J Natl Cancer Inst. 2015;107(7).
61. Russo GI, Regis F, Castelli T, Favilla V, Privitera S, Giardina R, et al. A systematic review and meta-analysis of the diagnostic accuracy of prostate health index and 4-kallikrein panel score in predicting overall and high-grade prostate cancer. Clin Genitourin Cancer. 2017;15(4):429–39e1.
62. Vickers A, Vertosick EA, Sjoberg DD, Roobol MJ, Hamdy F, Neal D, et al. Properties of the 4-Kallikrein panel outside the diagnostic gray zone: meta-analysis of patients with positive digital rectal examination or prostate specific antigen 10 ng/ml and above. J Urol. 2017;197(3 Pt 1):607–13.
63. Punnen S, Nahar B, Prakash NS, Sjoberg DD, Zappala SM, Parekh DJ. The 4Kscore predicts the grade and stage of prostate cancer in the radical prostatectomy specimen: results from a multi-institutional prospective trial. Eur Urol Focus. 2017;3(1):94–9.
64. Carlsson S, Maschino A, Schroder F, Bangma C, Steyerberg EW, van der Kwast T, et al. Predictive value of four kallikrein markers for pathologically insignificant compared with aggressive prostate cancer in radical prostatectomy specimens: results from the European randomized study of screening for prostate cancer section Rotterdam. Eur Urol. 2013;64(5):693–9.
65. Bussemakers MJ, van Bokhoven A, Verhaegh GW, Smit FP, Karthaus HF, Schalken JA, et al. DD3: a new prostate-specific gene, highly overexpressed in prostate cancer. Cancer Res. 1999;59(23):5975–9.
66. Hessels D, Klein Gunnewiek JM, van Oort I, Karthaus HF, van Leenders GJ, van Balken B, et al. DD3(PCA3)-based molecular urine analysis for the diagnosis of prostate cancer. Eur Urol. 2003;44(1):8–15; discussion 6.
67. Carroll PR, Parsons JK, Andriole G, Bahnson RR, Castle EP, Catalona WJ, et al. NCCN guidelines insights: prostate cancer early detection, version 2.2016. J Natl Compr Canc Netw. 2016;14(5):509–19.
68. Marks LS, Fradet Y, Deras IL, Blase A, Mathis J, Aubin SM, et al. PCA3 molecular urine assay for prostate cancer in men undergoing repeat biopsy. Urology. 2007;69(3):532–5.
69. Haese A, de la Taille A, van Poppel H, Marberger M, Stenzl A, Mulders PF, et al. Clinical utility of the PCA3 urine assay in European men scheduled for repeat biopsy. Eur Urol. 2008;54(5):1081–8.
70. Wei JT, Feng Z, Partin AW, Brown E, Thompson I, Sokoll L, et al. Can urinary PCA3 supplement PSA in the early detection of prostate cancer? J Clin Oncol. 2014;32(36):4066–72.
71. Thompson IM, Ankerst DP, Chi C, Goodman PJ, Tangen CM, Lucia MS, et al. Assessing prostate cancer risk: results from the prostate cancer prevention trial. J Natl Cancer Inst. 2006;98(8):529–34.
72. Thompson IM Jr, Leach RJ, Ankerst DP. Focusing PSA testing on detection of high-risk prostate cancers by incorporating patient preferences into decision making. JAMA. 2014;312(10):995–6.
73. Roobol MJ, Steyerberg EW, Kranse R, Wolters T, van den Bergh RC, Bangma CH, et al. A risk-based strategy improves prostate-specific antigen-driven detection of prostate cancer. Eur Urol. 2010;57(1):79–85.
74. Foley RW, Maweni RM, Gorman L, Murphy K, Lundon DJ, Durkan G, et al. European randomised study of screening for prostate cancer (ERSPC) risk calculators significantly outperform the prostate cancer prevention trial (PCPT) 2.0 in the prediction of prostate cancer: a multi-institutional study. BJU Int. 2016;118(5):706–13.

75. Lundon DJ, Kelly BD, Foley R, Loeb S, Fitzpatrick JM, Watson RW, et al. Prostate cancer risk assessment tools in an unscreened population. World J Urol. 2015;33(6):827–32.
76. Foley RW, Lundon DJ, Murphy K, Murphy TB, Galvin DJ, Watson RW. Predicting prostate cancer: analysing the clinical efficacy of prostate cancer risk calculators in a referral population. Ir J Med Sci. 2015;184(3):701–6.
77. Kattan MW, Eastham JA, Stapleton AM, Wheeler TM, Scardino PT. A preoperative nomogram for disease recurrence following radical prostatectomy for prostate cancer. J Natl Cancer Inst. 1998;90(10):766–71.
78. Kattan MW, Wheeler TM, Scardino PT. Postoperative nomogram for disease recurrence after radical prostatectomy for prostate cancer. J Clin Oncol. 1999;17(5):1499–507.
79. Kattan MW, Zelefsky MJ, Kupelian PA, Cho D, Scardino PT, Fuks Z, et al. Pretreatment nomogram that predicts 5-year probability of metastasis following three-dimensional conformal radiation therapy for localized prostate cancer. J Clin Oncol. 2003;21(24):4568–71.
80. Kattan MW, Zelefsky MJ, Kupelian PA, Scardino PT, Fuks Z, Leibel SA. Pretreatment nomogram for predicting the outcome of three-dimensional conformal radiotherapy in prostate cancer. J Clin Oncol. 2000;18(19):3352–9.
81. Kattan MW, Potters L, Blasko JC, Beyer DC, Fearn P, Cavanagh W, et al. Pretreatment nomogram for predicting freedom from recurrence after permanent prostate brachytherapy in prostate cancer. Urology. 2001;58(3):393–9.
82. Bjurlin MA, Meng X, Le Nobin J, Wysock JS, Lepor H, Rosenkrantz AB, et al. Optimization of prostate biopsy: the role of magnetic resonance imaging targeted biopsy in detection, localization and risk assessment. J Urol. 2014;192(3):648–58.
83. Meng X, Rosenkrantz AB, Mendhiratta N, Fenstermaker M, Huang R, Wysock JS, et al. Relationship between prebiopsy multiparametric magnetic resonance imaging (MRI), biopsy indication, and MRI-ultrasound fusion-targeted prostate biopsy outcomes. Eur Urol. 2016;69(3):512–7.
84. Liddell H, Jyoti R, Haxhimolla HZ. mp-MRI prostate characterised PIRADS 3 lesions are associated with a low risk of clinically significant prostate cancer—a retrospective review of 92 biopsied PIRADS 3 lesions. Curr Urol. 2015;8(2):96–100.
85. Kuru TH, Roethke MC, Rieker P, Roth W, Fenchel M, Hohenfellner M, et al. Histology core-specific evaluation of the European Society of Urogenital Radiology (ESUR) standardised scoring system of multiparametric magnetic resonance imaging (mpMRI) of the prostate. BJU Int. 2013;112(8):1080–7.
86. NiMhurchu E, O'Kelly F, Murphy IG, Lavelle LP, Collins CD, Lennon G, et al. Predictive value of PI-RADS classification in MRI-directed transrectal ultrasound guided prostate biopsy. Clin Radiol. 2016;71(4):375–80.
87. Park SY, Jung DC, Oh YT, Cho NH, Choi YD, Rha KH, et al. Prostate cancer: PI-RADS version 2 helps preoperatively predict clinically significant cancers. Radiology. 2016;280(1):108–16.
88. Martorana E, Pirola GM, Scialpi M, Micali S, Iseppi A, Bonetti LR, et al. Lesion volume predicts prostate cancer risk and aggressiveness: validation of its value alone and matched with prostate imaging reporting and data system score. BJU Int. 2017;120(1):92–103.
89. Min JH, Park BK, Park JJ, Park SY, Kim CK. Preoperative assessment of prostate cancer using prebiopsy MRI. AJR Am J Roentgenol. 2014;203(2):341–6.
90. Bjurlin MA, Taneja SS. Prediagnostic risk assessment with prostate MRI and MRI-targeted biopsy. Urol Clin North Am. 2017;44(4):535–46.
91. Mertan FV, Greer MD, Shih JH, George AK, Kongnyuy M, Muthigi A, et al. Prospective evaluation of the prostate imaging reporting and data system version 2 for prostate cancer detection. J Urol. 2016;196(3):690–6.
92. Borofsky MS, Rosenkrantz AB, Abraham N, Jain R, Taneja SS. Does suspicion of prostate cancer on integrated T2 and diffusion-weighted MRI predict more adverse pathology on radical prostatectomy? Urology. 2013;81(6):1279–83.
93. de Rooij M, Hamoen EH, Futterer JJ, Barentsz JO, Rovers MM. Accuracy of multiparametric MRI for prostate cancer detection: a meta-analysis. AJR Am J Roentgenol. 2014;202(2):343–51.

94. Giles SL, Morgan VA, Riches SF, Thomas K, Parker C, deSouza NM. Apparent diffusion coefficient as a predictive biomarker of prostate cancer progression: value of fast and slow diffusion components. AJR Am J Roentgenol. 2011;196(3):586–91.
95. Tamada T, Dani H, Taneja SS, Rosenkrantz AB. The role of whole-lesion apparent diffusion coefficient analysis for predicting outcomes of prostate cancer patients on active surveillance. Abdom Radiol (NY). 2017;42(9):2340–5.
96. van As NJ, de Souza NM, Riches SF, Morgan VA, Sohaib SA, Dearnaley DP, et al. A study of diffusion-weighted magnetic resonance imaging in men with untreated localised prostate cancer on active surveillance. Eur Urol. 2009;56(6):981–7.
97. De Cobelli F, Ravelli S, Esposito A, Giganti F, Gallina A, Montorsi F, et al. Apparent diffusion coefficient value and ratio as noninvasive potential biomarkers to predict prostate cancer grading: comparison with prostate biopsy and radical prostatectomy specimen. AJR Am J Roentgenol. 2015;204(3):550–7.
98. Henderson DR, de Souza NM, Thomas K, Riches SF, Morgan VA, Sohaib SA, et al. Nine-year follow-up for a study of diffusion-weighted magnetic resonance imaging in a prospective prostate cancer active surveillance cohort. Eur Urol. 2016;69(6):1028–33.
99. Lee H, Kim CK, Park BK, Sung HH, Han DH, Jeon HG, et al. Accuracy of preoperative multiparametric magnetic resonance imaging for prediction of unfavorable pathology in patients with localized prostate cancer undergoing radical prostatectomy. World J Urol. 2017;35(6):929–34.
100. Park JJ, Kim CK, Park SY, Park BK, Lee HM, Cho SW. Prostate cancer: role of pretreatment multiparametric 3-T MRI in predicting biochemical recurrence after radical prostatectomy. AJR Am J Roentgenol. 2014;202(5):W459–65.
101. Yoon MY, Park J, Cho JY, Jeong CW, Ku JH, Kim HH, et al. Predicting biochemical recurrence in patients with high-risk prostate cancer using the apparent diffusion coefficient of magnetic resonance imaging. Investig Clin Urol. 2017;58(1):12–9.
102. Kim TH, Kim CK, Park BK, Jeon HG, Jeong BC, Seo SI, et al. Relationship between Gleason score and apparent diffusion coefficients of diffusion-weighted magnetic resonance imaging in prostate cancer patients. Can Urol Assoc J. 2016;10(11–12):E377–E82.
103. Niu XK, He WF, Zhang Y, Das SK, Li J, Xiong Y, et al. Developing a new PI-RADS v2-based nomogram for forecasting high-grade prostate cancer. Clin Radiol. 2017;72(6):458–64.
104. Fang D, Zhao C, Ren D, Yu W, Wang R, Wang H, et al. Could magnetic resonance imaging help to identify the presence of prostate cancer before initial biopsy? The development of nomogram predicting the outcomes of prostate biopsy in the Chinese population. Ann Surg Oncol. 2016;23(13):4284–92.
105. Bjurlin MA SS, Venkataraman R, Mendhiratta N, Meng X, Rosenkrantz AB, Huang WC, Lepor H, Taneja SS. Prediction of prostate cancer risk among men undergoing combined MRI-targeted and systematic biopsy using novel pre-biopsy nomograms that incorporate MRI findings. Urology. 2017.
106. Decoster L, Van Puyvelde K, Mohile S, Wedding U, Basso U, Colloca G, et al. Screening tools for multidimensional health problems warranting a geriatric assessment in older cancer patients: an update on SIOG recommendationsdagger. Ann Oncol. 2015;26(2):288–300.
107. Extermann M, Aapro M, Bernabei R, Cohen HJ, Droz JP, Lichtman S, et al. Use of comprehensive geriatric assessment in older cancer patients: recommendations from the task force on CGA of the International Society of Geriatric Oncology (SIOG). Crit Rev Oncol Hematol. 2005;55(3):241–52.
108. Puts MT, Hardt J, Monette J, Girre V, Springall E, Alibhai SM. Use of geriatric assessment for older adults in the oncology setting: a systematic review. J Natl Cancer Inst. 2012;104(15):1133–63.
109. Wildiers H, Heeren P, Puts M, Topinkova E, Janssen-Heijnen ML, Extermann M, et al. International Society of Geriatric Oncology consensus on geriatric assessment in older patients with cancer. J Clin Oncol. 2014;32(24):2595–603.

110. Droz JP, Albrand G, Gillessen S, Hughes S, Mottet N, Oudard S, et al. Management of Prostate Cancer in elderly patients: recommendations of a task force of the International Society of Geriatric Oncology. Eur Urol. 2017;72(4):521–31.
111. Soubeyran P, Bellera C, Goyard J, Heitz D, Cure H, Rousselot H, et al. Screening for vulnerability in older cancer patients: the ONCODAGE prospective multicenter cohort study. PLoS One. 2014;9(12):e115060.
112. Borson S, Scanlan JM, Chen PJ, Ganguli M. The mini-cog as a screen for dementia: validation in a population-based sample. J Am Geriatr Soc. 2003;51(10):1451–4.
113. Powsner S, Powsner D. Cognition, copyright, and the classroom. Am J Psychiatry. 2005;162(3):627–8.
114. Tsoi KK, Chan JY, Hirai HW, Wong SY, Kwok TC. Cognitive tests to detect dementia: a systematic review and meta-analysis. JAMA Intern Med. 2015;175(9):1450–8.
115. Mendhiratta N, Rosenkrantz AB, Meng X, Wysock JS, Fenstermaker M, Huang R, et al. Magnetic resonance imaging-ultrasound fusion targeted prostate biopsy in a consecutive cohort of men with no previous biopsy: reduction of over detection through improved risk stratification. J Urol. 2015;194(6):1601–6.
116. Fenstermaker M, Mendhiratta N, Bjurlin MA, Meng X, Rosenkrantz AB, Huang R, et al. Risk stratification by urinary prostate cancer gene 3 testing before magnetic resonance imaging-ultrasound fusion-targeted prostate biopsy among men with no history of biopsy. Urology. 2017;99:174–9.

Chapter 3
Utilizing Biomarkers in Patients with Prior Negative Prostate Biopsy

James T. Kearns and Daniel W. Lin

Clinical Case Scenario: A 64-year-old man with a PSA of 7.5 and a previous negative biopsy whose PSA rises to 10 in a year and wants to utilize markers as opposed to repeat imaging and/or biopsy and wants a recommendation.

We are presented with a 64-year-old man who has a rising PSA from 7.5 ng/mL to 10 ng/mL over a 1-year period. He has a history of one prior negative prostate biopsy 2 years ago, and he has not previously been diagnosed with prostate cancer. He specifically states that he would prefer to use biomarkers to better understand his risk of having prostate cancer prior to undergoing a repeat biopsy. He has no urinary voiding symptoms or pelvic discomfort, and he has no family history of prostate cancer.

Biomarkers have been defined as, "a characteristic that is objectively measured and evaluated as an indicator of normal biological processes, pathogenic processes, or pharmacologic responses to a therapeutic intervention." [1] Importantly, biomarkers are, at best, surrogate end points when they are carefully validated and properly applied, and they are not actual end points of disease, such as metastasis or death [2]. The characteristics of an ideal biomarker are listed in Table 3.1.

Biomarkers in prostate cancer can be used at multiple timepoints in the course of the disease to predict various outcomes. Prior to diagnosis, biomarkers can help

J. T. Kearns, M.D. (✉)
Department of Urology, University of Washington, Seattle, WA, USA
e-mail: jkearns1@uw.edu

D. W. Lin, M.D.
Department of Urology, University of Washington, Seattle, WA, USA

Division of Public Health Sciences, Fred Hutchinson Cancer Research Center, Seattle, WA, USA

© Springer International Publishing AG, part of Springer Nature 2018
S. S. Chang, M. S. Cookson (eds.), *Prostate Cancer*,
https://doi.org/10.1007/978-3-319-78646-9_3

Table 3.1 Characteristics of
an ideal biomarker

Ideal biomarker characteristics
Sensitive and specific for disease processes
Correlates with disease outcome
Reproducible
Quick and easy assay
Low cost
Source biospecimen easily collected

stratify risk of a prostate cancer diagnosis or, more specifically, a high-risk prostate cancer diagnosis. After the initial diagnosis, biomarkers may help stratify the risk of harboring more aggressive prostate cancer at radical prostatectomy and/or may aid in understanding the underlying aggressiveness beyond the clinical information. Following primary treatment or at time of disease progression, other biomarkers can provide prognostic information regarding the likelihood of recurrence, metastasis, or even death from prostate cancer.

Given the wide variety of available biomarkers and the information that they provide, it is imperative to understand what questions the biomarkers are attempting to answer and how well that they can provide that information. Biomarkers are evaluated by a variety of statistical measures, such as sensitivity, specificity, negative and positive predictive value, and accuracy for their various end points. In the case of our patient, he is in the pre-diagnosis state, and he has undergone a previous prostate biopsy. He wishes to avoid an unnecessary biopsy in the future while minimizing his risk of missing a diagnosis of prostate cancer that may require treatment. Given this scenario, perhaps the most important information that a biomarker can provide in this instance is the negative predictive value (NPV) for diagnosis of prostate cancer. Perhaps even more important is the NPV for high-grade disease, a more clinically relevant end point with the knowledge that most low-risk patients can be managed safely with active surveillance. Patients in these clinical situations often want assurance regarding the decision to avoid biopsy. At the same time, patients will likely accept a biopsy if it seems that their chances of harboring cancer are high or if we cannot predict that they *do not* have cancer with enough certainty (i.e., high NPV).

Current Clinical Information

Prior to evaluating the impact of biomarkers on our patient's risk of having cancer, we must first understand his risk for having cancer without using additional biomarkers. In other words, with the available clinical information (e.g., PSA, age, digital rectal examination (DRE), previous biopsy status, family history), what is his predicted risk of harboring prostate cancer and how might a biomarker improve upon that prediction? Both the Prostate Cancer Prevention Trial [3] (PCPT) and European Randomized Screening for Prostate Cancer Trial [4] (ERSPC) have previously published calculators predicting the risk of a patient harboring prostate cancer. According to the PCPT, our patient has an 11% chance of having high-grade prostate cancer, a 15% chance of having low-grade prostate cancer, and a 74% chance of having no cancer on repeat biopsy. In the same patient, the ERSPC estimates that our patient has a 13% chance of having any cancer on biopsy and a 3% chance of having "significant" cancer (defined as ≥ T2b and/or Gleason ≥ 7). Each calculator relies on different clinical information to inform their models, but they both take into account that this patient has undergone a previous negative biopsy and that his PSA is 10. Additionally, there is a report by ElShafei et al. [5] suggesting that our patient would be more likely to have less aggressive disease at prostatectomy than a man diagnosed on a first biopsy. Finally, the rise in PSA from 7.5 ng/mL to 10 ng/mL over the course of 1 year represents an increase of 2.5 ng/mL/year. This is greater than the cutoff of 0.75 ng/mL/year proposed by Carter and Person [6] as putting our patient at higher risk of harboring prostate cancer. Most risk calculators and nomograms do not take into account the rate of rise, i.e., PSA kinetics, as part of the prediction.

In sum, we have a patient who has a 13–26% chance of having any prostate cancer, and a 3–11% chance of having significant prostate cancer on repeat biopsy, according to the readily available PCPT and ERSPC calculators. His risk is further modified by his history of previous negative prostate biopsy (decreased risk of significant disease) and his increasing PSA at a rate of 2.5 ng/mL/year (increased risk of having cancer). The question we now face is, can biomarkers help our patient make a more informed and certain decision about whether or not to proceed with prostate biopsy? Herein, we will turn to a discussion of available biomarkers to aid in this clinical scenario.

Free PSA

Prostate-specific antigen exists in two forms in the blood, unbound PSA (or "free PSA") or complexed PSA (with α1-antichymotrypsin and α2-macroglobulin) [7]. Christensson et al. [8] found that free PSA (fPSA) constituted a significantly smaller fraction of overall serum PSA in men with prostate cancer than those with benign prostatic hyperplasia (BPH). Given this finding, it was hypothesized that the %fPSA may aid diagnostic accuracy of PSA screening.

Catalona and colleagues [9] prospectively evaluated the utility of %fPSA to predict diagnosis of prostate cancer in men aged 50–75 years with serum PSA levels between 4.0 and 10.0 ng/mL. In this study population, they found that increasing %fPSA was significantly correlated with decreased probability of prostate cancer diagnosis. Men with a %fPSA <10% had a 56% chance of having prostate cancer on biopsy, compared with 8% of men having prostate cancer when their fPSA % was greater than 25%. Partin and colleagues [10] similarly evaluated 246 men at two centers, finding that the mean %fPSA was 14.1 ± 6.4 in men with cancer versus 18.2 ± 9.1 in men without cancer. They found that in men with a PSA between 4.0 and 10.0 ng/mL, a 95% sensitivity and 20% specificity could be obtained with a

%fPSA cutoff of 25%. Thus, prostate biopsies could be avoided in 20% of men while maintaining a 95% sensitivity. The authors did not report either a PPV or NPV for a 25% fPSA cutoff. Ankerst et al. [11] retrospectively reviewed 79 men in the San Antonio Biomarkers of Risk trial who received prostate biopsy for a PSA > 4.0 ng/mL and were found not to have cancer. They found that 25/79 men (31.6%) would have avoided a biopsy by using a %fPSA threshold of 25% to prompt a biopsy. Catalona and colleagues [12] evaluated whether %fPSA better predicted presence of prostate cancer in men with prior negative prostate biopsy in a cohort of 99 men. While the authors do not present an NPV for %fPSA, they found that using a %fPSA cutoff of 30% would detect 95% of cancers while avoiding 12% of biopsies. Taken together, %fPSA may help stratify risk of initial prostate cancer diagnosis, but its use in men with prior negative biopsy is less well defined.

Prostate Health Index

The Prostate Health Index (phi) incorporates multiple isoforms of PSA with the goal of improving specificity for prostate cancer diagnosis. The isoform [−2] proPSA is the primary form of fPSA in prostate cancer tissue, and PHI is calculated as $\left(\left([-2] proPSA / fPSA \right) \times \sqrt{PSA} \right)$ [13]. Catalona and colleagues [13] evaluated 892 men with no history of prostate cancer, normal rectal examination, serum PSA 2–10 ng/mL, and a ≥ 6-core prostate biopsy. They found that phi was significantly more specific for detection of prostate cancer and Gleason ≥7 prostate cancer. The AUC for phi was 0.703 for detection of prostate cancer and 0.724 for detection of Gleason ≥4 + 3 prostate cancer, which was significantly better than fPSA and total PSA (tPSA). In the subset of 658 men with PSA between 4 and 10 ng/mL, Loeb and collaborators [14] found that phi had an AUC of 0.708 for detection of prostate cancer and 0.707 for detection of Gleason ≥7 prostate cancer. With a 90% sensitivity cutoff (phi < 28.6), 30.1% of patients could be spared an unnecessary biopsy for no or insignificant cancer. A nomogram generated from this patient population to predict diagnosis of Gleason ≥7 prostate cancer using phi had an AUC of 0.746 [15]. Using a phi value of 35, the NPV for aggressive prostate cancer was 95%, and it increased to 96.8% at a phi cutoff of 28.

Lazzeri et al. [16] reviewed 222 men with prior negative prostate biopsies to assess if phi could improve decision-making regarding further biopsy. They found that phi outperformed %fPSA as a predictor of prostate cancer diagnosis. In total, 71 of 222 (31.9%) patients had prostate cancer on repeat biopsy. Using a phi cutoff of 28.8 would have avoided a biopsy in 116 (52.3%) of men while missing 6/71 (8.4%) of diagnoses. None of the missed diagnoses would have been Gleason ≥7. The NPV for prostate cancer diagnosis was 84.4% at a phi cutoff of 28.8. Boegemann and colleagues [17] also examined 769 men ≤65 years with a PSA of 2–10 ng/mL. Of these men, 391 had at least 1 prior negative prostate biopsy. They found that the AUC for phi was 0.73 at initial biopsy and 0.74 at repeat biopsy for detection of prostate cancer, supporting the performance of phi for both the initial and repeat biopsy population.

Kallikrein Panel (4Kscore)

The 4Kscore consists of a model incorporating 4-kallikrein forms (tPSA, fPSA, intact PSA, and human kallikrein 2 [hK2]) in addition to digital rectal examination, prior biopsy status, and age. The 4Kscore reports the specific probability of finding high-grade disease at the time of biopsy. The 4Kscore is the actual PPV for high-grade disease; thus the NPV is 1–4Kscore. Various cut points for 4Kscore have been reported, and ultimately, the choice to proceed with biopsy is individualized to the acceptable risk that the patient and provider decide. Vickers et al. [18] developed this score using the Swedish arm of the ERSPC trial, consisting of 740 men who were biopsied for a PSA $\geq$ 3.0 ng/mL. The AUCs for any cancer and high-grade cancer in the 4Kscore were 0.836 and 0.903, respectively. When using a 20% threshold for cancer diagnosis, 60% of biopsies could have been avoided while missing 17% of all cancer diagnoses and 3% of high-grade cancers. This analysis was repeated on 2914 men in the overall ERSPC cohort [19]. The AUC for detection of cancer was 0.776 and for detection of high-grade cancer was 0.837. Using a 20% risk threshold, 51.3% of biopsies could be avoided while missing 24% of cancers overall and 12% of high-grade cancers.

A multiinstitutional study in the United States published by Parekh et al. [20] evaluated the 4Kscore in 1012 men who were scheduled for prostate biopsy of which 139 had a previous negative biopsy. They found an AUC of 0.821 for diagnosis of Gleason $\geq$7 prostate cancer in all men, but they did not present a subgroup analysis of men with previous negative biopsy. Using a risk threshold of 6% (NPV = 0.94), 30% of biopsies could have been avoided in this population while missing 5% of Gleason $\geq$7 prostate cancers.

Bryant et al. [21] evaluated the predictive ability of the 4-kallikreins to predict the presence of prostate cancer and high-grade prostate cancer in 4765 men in the ProtecT trial. Given their different patient population, the authors generated a unique prediction model, rather than using the commercial 4Kscore. They found that the model incorporating all 4-kallikreins had an AUC of 0.719 for prediction of prostate cancer and 0.820 for prediction of high-grade prostate cancer. This compared with values of 0.634 and 0.738 for PSA alone for prediction of any prostate cancer or high-grade prostate cancer. Using a risk cutoff for high-grade prostate cancer of 6% (the lowest risk threshold for any diagnosis presented was 20%), 43% of prostate biopsies could be avoided while missing 11% of high-grade cancers. Gupta and colleagues [22] evaluated the 4Kscore in patients in 925 men in the Rotterdam arm of the ERSPC with a PSA $\geq$ 3.0 ng/mL and a previous negative prostate biopsy. The AUCs for detection of any cancer and Gleason $\geq$7 cancer were 0.681 and 0.873, respectively. Using a 10% risk threshold (the lowest presented by the authors) for deciding to proceed with repeat biopsy would avoid 54% of biopsies while missing 31% of cancer diagnoses and 5% of high-grade cancers.

Nordstrom et al. [23] compared the predictive ability of the 4-kallikrein panel and phi in a population of 531 men undergoing first-time prostate biopsy for a PSA between 3 and 15 ng/mL. They found that the 4-kallikrein panel had AUCs of 0.690 and 0.718 for prediction of any-grade and high-grade prostate cancer, compared with AUCs of 0.704 and 0.711 for phi. Both the 4-kallikrein panel and phi outperformed PSA alone. In addition, the authors state that the results were similar in sensitivity analyses including men with a previous biopsy, but they do not provide the data. Taken together, the predictive abilities of the 4Kscore and phi are not significantly different.

Prostate Cancer Antigen 3 (PCA3)

Prostate cancer antigen 3 (PCA3) was initially reported by Bussemakers and colleagues [24] as a noncoding mRNA that is highly overexpressed in prostate cancer. Importantly, PCA3 is not related to prostate volume (unlike PSA) and is directly associated with grade and volume of prostate cancer [25]. Marks et al. [26] initially presented PCA3 as a urine biomarker for prediction of prostate cancer on repeat biopsy. The authors evaluated 233 men with PSA $\geq$ 2.5 ng/mL and at least one negative biopsy. Urine was collected after an attentive digital rectal examination (three strokes per lobe). They found that the AUC for PCA3 was 0.68, compared with 0.52 for PSA. At a PCA3 score cutoff of 35, the sensitivity and specificity for prediction of prostate cancer were 0.58 and 0.72, respectively. With a PCA3 score $\leq$ 5, the probability of diagnosing prostate cancer was 12%, compared with 50% for a PCA3 score > 100. These findings were confirmed by Haese and collaborators [27] in a cohort of 463 European men with one or two previous negative prostate biopsies. The AUC for prediction of prostate cancer was 0.658, compared with 0.578 for %fPSA. With a PCA3 score cutoff of 35, the sensitivity was 0.47, and the specificity was 0.72. With a PCA3 score $\leq$ 5, the probability of diagnosing prostate cancer was 12%, compared with 47% for a PCA3 score > 100. Negative predictive values were not reported in these studies.

Deras and colleagues [25] evaluated the effectiveness of PCA3 in predicting prostate cancer in 570 men. They found that the AUC for prediction of prostate cancer was 0.70 in men without previous biopsy (277 men) and 0.68 in men (280) with previous negative biopsy. Aubin et al. [28] evaluated the PCA3 score in men with previous negative biopsy in the placebo arm of the REDUCE trial. In their analysis of 1072 men, the AUC for prediction of prostate cancer was 0.693, versus 0.612 for serum PSA. In a logistic regression model including PCA3 score, age, family history, %fPSA, prostate volume, and serum PSA, the AUC for prediction of prostate cancer was 0.753. Gittelman and collaborators [29] similarly evaluated 466 men with a least 1 prior negative prostate biopsy for the effectiveness of PCA3 score in predicting the presence of prostate cancer. The negative predictive value for detection of prostate cancer at a PCA3 score cutoff of 25 was 90%. In a pivotal prospective trial by the NCI Early Detection Research Network (EDRN), Wei et al. [30] reported that the NPV for a PCA3 cut point of 20 in men with previous negative biopsy was 88%. Taken together, in our clinical scenario, we can tell the patient that he has an approximate 90% chance of a negative biopsy if his PCA3 is <20.

DNA Methylation Assays (ConfirmMDx)

DNA methylation is an example of an epigenetic aberration that has been well established as an early molecular alteration in prostate cancer oncogenesis. For example, GSTP1 methylation occurs in up to 90% of prostate cancer cases and has been validated in multiple studies [31]. ConfirmMDx is a commercial assay designed to evaluate tissue from previous negative prostate biopsies for DNA methylation as a biomarker for false negative prostate biopsy. This assay measures methylation of three markers, *GSTP1*, *APC*, and *RASSF1*, on histologically negative prostate tissue and reveals areas within the prostate that harbor methylation signatures which suggest occult prostate cancer. The MATLOC study [32] published by Stewart et al. tested archived prostate biopsy samples in 498 subjects who subsequently underwent prostate biopsy. They found that this assay had an NPV of 90% for prediction of prostate cancer, and all patients who had Gleason ≥7 prostate cancer had at a positive assay. The DOCUMENT multicenter trial [33] in the United States, authored by Partin and colleagues, evaluated the same assay on 350 men from 5 centers, all of whom had a negative biopsy followed by another prostate biopsy within 24 months. They found that the NPV for cancer on subsequent biopsy was 88% in their population. Van Neste et al. [34] pooled the results from both of the prior studies to generate a risk score from the DNA methylation results, namely, the EpiScore. These investigators reported that the EpiScore had an NPV of 96% for the prediction of Gleason ≥7 prostate cancer. This score has not yet been validated in an external cohort. Taken together, in our clinical scenario, we can tell the patient that he has an approximate 88–90% chance of a negative biopsy if his ConfirmMDx is negative and a 96% chance of not finding Gleason ≥7 prostate cancer if his EpiScore is negative.

Current Guidelines and Future Directions

Multiple professional societies have made recommendations regarding advanced testing in the face of rising PSA after previous negative prostate biopsy. The National Comprehensive Cancer Network (NCCN) states that %fPSA, phi, urine PCA3, 4Kscore, and ConfirmMDx are all options to further risk stratify patients [35]. Similarly the European Association of Urology (EAU) states that urine PCA3, 4Kscore, and ConfirmMDx may help with decision-making after negative biopsy

[35]. The American Urological Association (AUA) does not make specific recommendations for men with prior negative biopsy [36]. The EAU further has non-biomarker-based recommendations for repeat biopsy, the tests, substrates, molecular signal, FDA approval status, and performance characteristics for biomarkers after previous negative biopsy [35].

Summary

In the clinical scenario of a persistently elevated PSA with a prior negative biopsy, the aforementioned studies clearly demonstrate the additional predictive abilities of numerous biomarkers that add additional value above and beyond PSA combined with available clinical metrics. Future studies should focus specifically on the detection of high-grade prostate cancer, cost-effectiveness of widescale implementation, and incorporation of biomarkers into multinomial predictive tools or calculators. Additionally, although our patient was specifically interested in biomarkers, the emerging imaging platforms (e.g., multiparametric MRI) will need to be integrated within the biomarker domain with perhaps a low-cost biomarker serving as a trigger for advanced imaging as has been suggested by others [37]. At this point for our patient, in alignment with established guidelines, we would recommend consideration of one of the biomarkers with particular attention to the high NPV for detection of prostate cancer at next biopsy.

References

1. Biomarkers Definitions Working Group. Biomarkers and surrogate endpoints: preferred definitions and conceptual framework. Clin Pharmacol Ther. 2001;69:89–95.
2. Strimbu K, Tavel JA. What are biomarkers? Curr Opin HIV AIDS. 2010;5:463–6.
3. Thompson IM, et al. Assessing prostate cancer risk: results from the prostate cancer prevention trial. J Natl Cancer Inst. 2006;98:529–34.
4. Roobol MJ, et al. A risk-based strategy improves prostate-specific antigen–driven detection of prostate cancer. Eur Urol. 2010;57:79–85.
5. ElShafei A, et al. More favorable pathological outcomes in men with low risk prostate cancer diagnosed on repeat versus initial Transrectal ultrasound guided prostate biopsy. J Urol. 2016;195:1767–72.
6. Carter HB, Pearson JD. Prostate-specific antigen velocity and repeated measures of prostate-specific antigen. Urol Clin North Am. 1997;24:333–8.
7. Christensson A, Laurell C-B, Lilja H. Enzymatic activity of prostate-specific antigen and its reactions with extracellular serine proteinase inhibitors. Eur J Biochem. 1990;194:755–63.
8. Christensson A, et al. Serum prostate specific antigen complexed to α1-antichymotrypsin as an indicator of prostate cancer. J Urol. 1993;150:100–5.
9. Catalona WJ, et al. Use of the percentage of free prostate-specific antigen to enhance differentiation of prostate cancer from benign prostatic disease: a prospective multicenter clinical trial. JAMA. 1998;279:1542–7.

10. Partin AW, et al. Prospective evaluation of percent free-PSA and complexed-PSA for early detection of prostate cancer. Prostate Cancer Prostatic Dis. 1998;1:197–203.
11. Ankerst DP, et al. Serial percent-free PSA in combination with PSA for population-based early detection of prostate cancer. J Urol. 2016;196:355–60.
12. Catalona WJ, Beiser JA, Smith DS. Serum free prostate specific antigen and prostate specific antigen density measurements for predicting cancer in men with prior negative prostatic biopsies. J Urol. 1997;158:2162–7.
13. Catalona WJ, et al. A multi-center study of [−2]pro-prostate-specific antigen (PSA) in Combination with PSA and free PSA for prostate cancer detection in the 2.0 to 10.0 ng/mL PSA range. J Urol. 2011;185:1650–5.
14. Loeb S, et al. The prostate Health Index selectively identifies clinically significant prostate cancer. J Urol. 2015;193:1163–9.
15. Loeb S, et al. Prostate Health Index improves multivariable risk prediction of aggressive prostate cancer. BJU Int. 2017;120:61–8.
16. Lazzeri M, et al. Serum Index test %[−2]proPSA and prostate Health Index are more accurate than prostate specific antigen and %fPSA in predicting a positive repeat prostate biopsy. J Urol. 2012;188:1137–43.
17. Boegemann M, et al. The percentage of prostate-specific antigen (PSA) isoform [−2]proPSA and the prostate Health Index improve the diagnostic accuracy for clinically relevant prostate cancer at initial and repeat biopsy compared with total PSA and percentage free PSA in men aged ≤65 years. BJU Int. 2016;117:72–9.
18. Vickers AJ, et al. A panel of kallikrein markers can reduce unnecessary biopsy for prostate cancer: data from the European randomized study of prostate cancer screening in Göteborg, Sweden. BMC Med. 2008;6:19.
19. Vickers A, et al. Reducing unnecessary biopsy during prostate cancer screening using a four-Kallikrein panel: an independent replication. J Clin Oncol. 2010;28:2493–8.
20. Parekh DJ, et al. A multi-institutional prospective trial in the USA confirms that the 4Kscore accurately identifies men with high-grade prostate cancer. Eur Urol. 2015;68:464–70.
21. Bryant RJ, et al. Predicting high-grade cancer at ten-core prostate biopsy using four kallikrein markers measured in blood in the ProtecT study. J Natl Cancer Inst. 2015;107. https://doi.org/10.1093/jnci/djv095.
22. Gupta A, et al. A four-kallikrein panel for the prediction of repeat prostate biopsy: data from the European randomized study of prostate cancer screening in Rotterdam, Netherlands. Br J Cancer. 2010;103:708–14.
23. Nordström T, et al. Comparison between the four-kallikrein panel and prostate Health Index (PHI) for predicting prostate cancer. Eur Urol. 2015;68:139–46.
24. Bussemakers MJG, et al. DD3: a new prostate-specific Gene, highly overexpressed in prostate cancer. Cancer Res. 1999;59:5975–9.
25. Deras IL, et al. PCA3: a molecular urine assay for predicting prostate biopsy outcome. J Urol. 2008;179:1587–92.
26. Marks LS, et al. PCA3 molecular urine assay for prostate cancer in men undergoing repeat biopsy. Urology. 2007;69:532–5.
27. Haese A, et al. Clinical utility of the PCA3 urine assay in European men scheduled for repeat biopsy. Eur Urol. 2008;54:1081–8.
28. Aubin SMJ, et al. PCA3 molecular urine test for predicting repeat prostate biopsy outcome in populations at risk: validation in the placebo arm of the Dutasteride REDUCE trial. J Urol. 2010;184:1947–52.
29. Gittelman MC, et al. PCA3 molecular urine test as a predictor of repeat prostate biopsy outcome in men with previous negative biopsies: a prospective multicenter clinical study. J Urol. 2013;190:64–9.
30. Wei JT, et al. Can urinary PCA3 supplement PSA in the early detection of prostate cancer? J Clin Oncol. 2014;32:4066–72.

31. Van Neste L, et al. The epigenetic promise for prostate cancer diagnosis. Prostate. 2012;72:1248–61.
32. Stewart GD, et al. Clinical utility of an epigenetic assay to detect occult prostate cancer in histopathologically negative biopsies: results of the MATLOC study. J Urol. 2013;189:1110–6.
33. Partin AW, et al. Clinical validation of an epigenetic assay to predict negative histopathological results in repeat prostate biopsies. J Urol. 2014;192:1081–7.
34. Van Neste L, et al. Risk score predicts high-grade prostate cancer in DNA-methylation positive, histopathologically negative biopsies. Prostate. 2016;76:1078–87.
35. European Association of Urology. Prostate Cancer. Uroweb. 2014. http://uroweb.org/guideline/prostate-cancer/#5. Accessed 11 Oct 2017.
36. Carter HB, et al. Early detection of prostate cancer: AUA guideline. J Urol. 2013;190:419–26.
37. Leyten GHJM, et al. Value of PCA3 to predict biopsy outcome and its potential role in selecting patients for multiparametric MRI. Int J Mol Sci. 2013;14:11347–55.

Chapter 4
Active Surveillance in African-Americans

Samuel L. Washington III and Matthew R. Cooperberg

> **Clinical Case Scenario:** A 65-year-old healthy African-American man with a PSA of 4.8 ng/mL and a Gleason 3 + 3 prostate cancer found in a sextant biopsy.

In this case discussion, we will review the case of a healthy 65-year-old African-American (AA) man who was initially referred for further consultation and evaluation for an elevated prostate-specific antigen (PSA) level of 4.8 ng/mL. He stated he had no family history of prostate cancer. He denied urinary complaints or impaired erectile function. A smooth, enlarged gland was noted on digital rectal exam. Transrectal ultrasound of the prostate demonstrated a 50 mL prostate cancer with no hypoechoic lesions. A sextant biopsy was performed with pathology demonstrating Gleason 6 (3 + 3), Grade Group 1, adenocarcinoma of the prostate. One of ten cores contained cancer with approximately 20% core involvement. PSA density was 0.096. The patient reported that he has done his own reading about management of prostate cancer. He was also referred for consultation with a radiation oncologist but stated that he would prefer to avoid immediate surgery or radiation out of concern for side effects associated with each treatment option. He was most interested in active surveillance (AS), understanding it entails routine PSA testing and digital rectal exams. He understood AS does not always replace definitive treatment indefinitely but does reduce his risk of overtreatment.

S. L. Washington III, M.D. (✉) · M. R. Cooperberg, M.D., M.P.H.
Department of Urology, University of California, San Francisco, San Francisco, CA, USA
e-mail: Samuel.Washington@ucsf.edu; matthew.cooperberg@ucsf.edu

© Springer International Publishing AG, part of Springer Nature 2018
S. S. Chang, M. S. Cookson (eds.), *Prostate Cancer*,
https://doi.org/10.1007/978-3-319-78646-9_4

Evaluation and Guidelines

The American Urological Association/American Society for Radiation Oncology/ Society of Urologic Oncology (AUA/ASTRO/SUO) joint guideline for early detection of prostate cancer recommends that active surveillance (AS) be offered as the preferred option for most men with low-risk disease, following appropriate shared decision-making [1]. Prior to initiating AS, appropriate staging with a systematic prostate biopsy with transrectal ultrasound is required. The patient described above has a Cancer of the Prostate Risk Assessment (CAPRA) score of 1, and based on AUA and National Cancer Center Network (NCCN) risk stratification, he would be stratified as "very low" risk. By any risk stratification, he would meet eligibility criteria for AS based on his clinical and pathologic characteristics. The only extant national guideline focused specifically on AS was published by the American Society for Clinical Oncology (ASCO). Like the AUA/SUO/ASTRO guideline, the ASCO guideline endorses AS for most low-risk disease; it is the only guideline to mention race explicitly, cautioning that African-American men, like those with higher-volume disease or younger age at diagnosis, merit closer assessment at diagnosis to ensure that the cancer has not been under-sampled [2].

Racial Differences in Prostate Cancer Burden and Mortality

Prostate cancer is the most commonly diagnosed solid malignancy and the second most common cause of cancer-specific death for AA men [3]. Some have suggested that AA race alone confers higher risk disease and suggest caution offering AA men AS [4, 5]. The discussion of whether AS is appropriate stems from a known differential burden of high-risk prostate cancer and prostate cancer-specific mortality for AA men compared to white men. One such study showed that AA men faced a 2.2- to 3-fold higher rate of fatal cancer compared to white men despite overall rates of prostate cancer-specific mortality decreasing over the same interval. This disparity was particularly pronounced for younger men: AA men aged 45–49 faced 4.2-fold higher risk compared their white counterparts [6]. Partially due to this disparity, there continues to be a debate about the appropriateness of AS and the need to more accurately estimate risk for AA men [7–9].

The racial disparity gap in mortality is only partially explained by biological characteristics. One study evaluated racial disparity in prostate cancer mortality using SEER data, finding that tumor characteristics and comorbidities explained only half (54%) of the racial gap. They found that over half of the mortality gap is conditional on features identifiable after diagnosis [10]. Additional investigation has attempted to elucidate the roots of this well-established racial disparity, acknowledging these are most certainly multifactorial in nature. Known covariates such as marital status, health insurance, socioeconomic status, hospital characteristics, tumor stage/grade at diagnosis, and neighborhood characteristics can explain roughly half the observed disparity; how much of the remainder is explainable by inherited genetics, dietary and other environmental factors, and other unmeasured parameters remains unclear [11].

Should African American Men Be Eligible for Active Surveillance?

The basis for the caveat regarding the eligibility of AA men for AS in the ASCO guideline rests primarily on a 2013 study from the Johns Hopkins University radical prostatectomy cohort. In this cohort, 1801 men, including 256 AA men, met the restrictive NCCN "very low-risk" criteria before surgery. On multivariable analysis, the likelihood of adverse pathology defined by pGS $\geq 4 + 3$, pT3b, or pT3a with either positive margins or pGS $3 + 4$ was over threefold higher among AA men; as defined by CAPRA-S score ≥ 3, likelihood of adverse pathology was over sixfold higher among AA men [4]. A later study suggested that one explanation for higher rates of undersampling among AA men is a much higher proportion of anterior tumors, which are more frequently missed on standard transrectal ultrasound-guided biopsy [6]. Most recently, a follow-up study among a subset of 300 cases found distinct molecular subtypes by race but more importantly by location, with a higher proportion in particular of triple negative (ERG, SPINK1, and ETS-negative) tumors in the anterior zone [12].

As intriguing as these findings are, they have not been replicated in other contexts. A follow-up study including patients from both another large academic surgical cohort (University of California, San Francisco) and the Cancer of the Prostate Strategic Urologic Research Endeavor community-based registry found that neither upgrading nor upstaging was more common among AA vs. Caucasian men with low-risk disease at diagnosis, although rates of positive surgical margins were higher among AA men [13].

Furthermore, in a cohort based in the equal access healthcare United States Veteran Affairs system, a database with a much greater proportion of AA men than either of the prior studies, these differences in outcomes again were not confirmed. In this study again focusing on men with clinically low-risk prostate cancer, AA men were younger with higher PSA and PSA density compared to Caucasian men. However, AA race was not associated with pathologic upgrading, upstaging, nor positive surgical margins in multivariable logistic regression analyses. Similarly, race was not associated with time to biochemical recurrence after radical prostatectomy [14].

The explanation for these discrepant findings is not immediately clear. The relatively dramatic findings from the Johns Hopkins cohort may ultimately be a statistical fluke. Alternatively, it is possible that there are genetic and/or environmental characteristics unique to the AA population in and around Baltimore that are not representative of AA populations elsewhere in the country. Unfortunately, the studies mentioned above did not include sufficiently consistent data on anterior vs. posterior tumor location to validate the finding of location differences by race. In 2018, it seems reasonable to conclude, consistent with the ASCO guideline, that AA men should certainly be considered eligible for AS but also that relatively intense efforts to rule out undersampled high-risk disease (e.g., with MRI, genomic testing, and/or confirmatory biopsy specifically targeting the anterior zones) are particularly warranted in this group.

Considerations for Choosing Active Surveillance

In addition to assessing eligibility for AS, the question of whether AA men believe AS is appropriate should be considered. Racial concordance between physician and patient can improve perception of and satisfaction with care, but is not essential to good bilateral communication [15–17]. Mistrust in the healthcare system remains a reminder of past difficulties while race continues to impact treatment choice [18, 19]. Subsequently, race is significantly associated with reporting of decisional regret at 3 years after treatment in AA men with low- and intermediate-risk disease, and in fact race was the only factor positively associated with regret; however, regret was not statistically significantly less likely among AA men opting for AS vs. those undergoing active treatment [20]. A comprehensive approach to counseling, combined with acknowledgement of the patient's perspective, will facilitate utilization and optimized implementation of AS in this specific patient population. Given the possibly higher rates of undersampling among AA men, careful attention should be paid to consistency of follow-up among AA men, and to the extent that race associates with socioeconomic status and access to regular care, this concern is particularly salient in safety-net hospital settings [21].

Conclusions

Preferential adoption of AS as an alternative to immediate treatment for most men with low risk disease is a critical component of contemporary "smarter screening" approaches to prostate cancer early detection. While AA men were essentially unrepresented in the screening randomized trials, recent modeling studies do support the concept that AA men should receive particular attention in screening programs and potentially should start screening at an earlier age. An in-depth analysis from the CISNET group aimed to identify factors contributing to the disparity in prostate cancer mortality. AA men at all ages were noted to have a higher cumulative incidence of clinically significant disease despite observed disparities in PSA screening which increased with older ages. Multiple mathematical models predicted an increased risk of preclinical disease in AA men, contributing in turn to an increased risk of clinical diagnosis and of metastatic disease before diagnosis. On the other hand, risk of clinical disease after onset was similar between AA and the general population. These findings led the authors to conclude that AA men were at higher risk of preclinical and progressive prostate cancer, more likely to develop disease at younger ages and progress to metastasis before diagnosis. From these findings, the authors support earlier screening for AA men [22]. The SEER study described above likewise concluded that if AA men are at risk of more aggressive disease, they may benefit more from screening compared to white men [10].

Neither analysis, however, suggests that AA men diagnosed with what is confirmed to be low-risk disease should be managed differently from non-AA men. With appropriate counseling and risk stratification, AS remains an appropriate, and even preferred, management option for AA men. Future research is needed to determine to what extent AS protocols should be modified or intensified for AA men, and what additive role novel imaging and other biomarkers should play.

References

1. Sanda MG, Cadeddu JA, Kirkby E, et al. Clinically localized prostate cancer: AUA/ASTRO/SUO guideline. Part I: risk stratification, shared decision making, and care options. J Urol. 2017. https://doi.org/10.1016/j.juro.2017.11.095.
2. Chen RC, Rumble RB, Loblaw DA, et al. Active Surveillance for the Management of Localized Prostate Cancer (Cancer Care Ontario guideline): American Society of Clinical Oncology clinical practice guideline endorsement. J Clin Oncol. 2016;34(18):2182–90. https://doi.org/10.1200/JCO.2015.65.7759.
3. DeSantis CE, Siegel RL, Sauer AG, et al. Cancer statistics for African Americans, 2016: progress and opportunities in reducing racial disparities. CA Cancer J Clin. 2016;66(4):290–308. https://doi.org/10.3322/caac.21340.
4. Sundi D, Ross AE, Humphreys EB, et al. African American men with very low-risk prostate cancer exhibit adverse oncologic outcomes after radical prostatectomy: should active surveillance still be an option for them? J Clin Oncol. 2013;31(24):2991–7. https://doi.org/10.1200/JCO.2012.47.0302.
5. Sundi D, Kryvenko ON, Carter HB, Ross AE, Epstein JI, Schaeffer EM. Pathological examination of radical prostatectomy specimens in men with very low risk disease at biopsy reveals distinct zonal distribution of cancer in black American men. J Urol. 2014;191(1):60–7. https://doi.org/10.1016/j.juro.2013.06.021.
6. Kelly SP, Rosenberg PS, Anderson WF, et al. Trends in the incidence of fatal prostate cancer in the United States by race. Eur Urol. 2017;71(2):195–201. https://doi.org/10.1016/j.eururo.2016.05.011.
7. Porten SP, Richardson DA, Odisho AY, McAninch JW, Carroll PR, Cooperberg MR. Oncology: prostate/testis/penis/urethra disproportionate presentation of high risk prostate cancer in a safety net health system. J Urol. 2010;184(5):1931–6. https://doi.org/10.1016/j.juro.2010.06.116.
8. Schreiber D, Chhabra A, Rineer J, Weedon J, Schwartz DA. Population-based study of men with low-volume low-risk prostate cancer: does African-American race predict for more aggressive disease? Clin Genitourin Cancer. 2015;13(4):e259–64. https://doi.org/10.1016/j.clgc.2015.02.006.
9. Pietzak EJ, Van Arsdalen K, Patel K, Malkowicz SB, Wein AJ, Oncology GTJ. Impact of race on selecting appropriate patients for active surveillance with seemingly low-risk prostate cancer. Urology. 2015;85(2):436–41. https://doi.org/10.1016/j.urology.2014.09.065.

10. Taksler GB, Keating NL, Cutler DM. Explaining racial differences in prostate cancer mortality. Cancer. 2012;118(17):4280–9. https://doi.org/10.1002/cncr.27379.
11. Ellis L, Canchola AJ, Spiegel D, Ladabaum U, Haile R, Gomez SL. Racial and ethnic disparities in cancer survival: the contribution of tumor, sociodemographic, institutional, and neighborhood characteristics. J Clin Oncol. 2018;36(1):25–33. https://doi.org/10.1200/JCO.2017.74.2049.
12. Faisal FA, Sundi D, Tosoian JJ, et al. Racial variations in prostate cancer molecular subtypes and androgen receptor signaling reflect anatomic tumor location. Eur Urol. 2016;70(1):14–7. https://doi.org/10.1016/j.eururo.2015.09.031.
13. Jalloh M, Myers F, Cowan JE, Carroll PR, Cooperberg MR. Racial variation in prostate cancer upgrading and upstaging among men with low-risk clinical characteristics. Eur Urol. 2015;67(3):451–7. https://doi.org/10.1016/j.eururo.2014.03.026.
14. Leapman MS, Freedland SJ, Aronson WJ, et al. Pathological and biochemical outcomes among African-American and Caucasian men with low risk prostate cancer in the SEARCH database: implications for active surveillance candidacy. J Urol. 2016;196(5):1408–14. https://doi.org/10.1016/j.juro.2016.06.086.
15. Cooper LA, Roter DL, Johnson RL, Ford DE, Steinwachs DM, Powe NR. Patient-centered communication, ratings of care, and concordance of patient and physician race. Ann Intern Med. 2003;139(11):907–15.
16. Blanchard J, Nayar S, Lurie N. Patient–provider and patient–staff racial concordance and perceptions of mistreatment in the health care setting. J Gen Intern Med. 2007;22(8):1184–9. https://doi.org/10.1007/s11606-007-0210-8.
17. Saha S, Komaromy M, Koepsell TD, Bindman AB. Patient-physician racial concordance and the perceived quality and use of health care. Arch Intern Med. 1999;159(9):997–1004.
18. Moses KA, Paciorek AT, Penson DF, Carroll PR, Master VA. Impact of ethnicity on primary treatment choice and mortality in men with prostate cancer: data from CaPSURE. J Clin Oncol. 2010;28(6):1069–74. https://doi.org/10.1200/JCO.2009.26.2469.
19. Moses KA, Orom H, Brasel A, Gaddy J, Underwood W. Racial/ethnic differences in the relative risk of receipt of specific treatment among men with prostate cancer. Urol Oncol. 2016;34(9):415.e7–415.e12. https://doi.org/10.1016/j.urolonc.2016.04.002.
20. Hurwitz LM, Cullen J, Kim DJ, et al. Longitudinal regret after treatment for low- and intermediate-risk prostate cancer. Cancer. 2017;123(21):4252–8. https://doi.org/10.1002/cncr.30841.
21. Osterberg EC, Palmer NRA, Harris CR, et al. Outcomes of men on active surveillance for low-risk prostate cancer at a safety-net hospital. Urol Oncol. 2017;35:663.e9–e154.
22. Tsodikov A, Gulati R, de Carvalho TM, et al. Is prostate cancer different in black men? Answers from 3 natural history models. Cancer. 2017;123(12):2312–9. https://doi.org/10.1002/cncr.30687.

Chapter 5
Focal Therapy Versus Surveillance in Intermediate-Risk Cancer

Kelly L. Stratton and Daniel Parker

Clinmical Case Scenario: A 58-year-old man with a PSA of 2.5 ng/mL and a normal DRE undergoes a sextant biopsy revealing 1 of 12 cores positive (<20%) for GS 7 (3 + 4) prostate cancer desires active surveillance or focal therapy.

Prostate cancer screening requires a balance between the identification of life-threatening disease that may benefit from early detection and the avoidance of over-treatment for patients who are not at risk of disease progression. Many factors are considered when making these decisions for screening, resulting in the recommendation for shared decision-making between patient and physician. The balance between risk and benefit of treatment may be weighed against the potential to have adverse side effects from the desired therapy. To reduce overtreatment and balance the unlikelihood of disease progression, active surveillance has been offered to men with low- and intermediate-risk disease. However, up to a third of patients on active surveillance eventually undergo treatment. Further, repeated evaluations and prostate biopsies can have detrimental effects on patient's mental status and quality of life. The potential to treat patients selectively while the tumor is small and localized has led to the advent of focal therapy for prostate cancer. Although the disease is felt to be multifocal, the thought that cancer risk is attributable to an index lesion that can be identified on prostate imaging is the cornerstone of focal therapy efficacy.

K. L. Stratton, M.D. (✉) · D. Parker, M.D.
Department of Urology, Stephenson Cancer Center,
University of Oklahoma Health Sciences Center, Oklahoma City, OK, USA
e-mail: Kelly-Stratton@ouhsc.edu

© Springer International Publishing AG, part of Springer Nature 2018
S. S. Chang, M. S. Cookson (eds.), *Prostate Cancer*,
https://doi.org/10.1007/978-3-319-78646-9_5

The potential to reduce the concomitant risk of side effects, obviate the need for repeated prostate biopsies, and achieve a cancer-free state has made focal therapy an increasingly popular choice for men who are eligible for this treatment. This clinical scenario represents a young gentleman with a small focus of intermediate-risk disease. Having intact genitourinary function must be balanced with the potential to prevent later morbidity or mortality. Although this patient is a candidate for definitive local therapy, the use of active surveillance and focal therapy will be explored.

Screening

Prostate cancer is the most common non-cutaneous cancer in men. The risk of harboring prostate cancer is roughly proportional to a patient's age as a percentage [1]. In 2017, over 160,000 men will be diagnosed with prostate cancer [2]. However, the risk of prostate cancer mortality varies based on the aggressiveness of the disease. Low-risk prostate cancer, as described by D'Amico, included men with Gleason score 6 prostate cancer, PSA <10 ng/mL, and clinical stage T2a or less [3]. Intermediate-risk disease includes those with a PSA between 10 and 20, clinical stage T2b or less, or the highest Gleason score of 7. The updated NCCN guidelines for prostate cancer suggest that men with favorable intermediate-risk prostate cancer, defined as Gleason grade 3 predominate histology $(3 + 4 = 7)$ and percentage of positive biopsy cores <50%, may be candidates for active surveillance [4]. The patient in this scenario has clinical features consistent with favorable intermediate-risk prostate cancer. Further, most studies of intermediate-risk prostate cancer patients undergoing focal therapy suggest that Gleason $3 + 4 = 7$ prostate cancer is the most common intermediate-risk criteria [5].

Diagnosis

The Gleason grading system has stood the test of time. However, the degree of cancer aggressiveness is NOT proportional to the numerical increase from Grade 3 to Grade 4. Several studies have found that Gleason 3 disease lacks the molecular hallmarks of cancer [6]. This is supported by the findings that Gleason Score 6 cancers have not been identified in lymph node metastases [7]. Conversely, large volume Gleason 6 cancers are concerning due to the potential for occult higher risk prostate cancer [8]. Finally, small volume Gleason $3 + 4$ are considered favorable intermediate-risk prostate cancers and may be eligible for active surveillance. This spectrum of risk based on clinicopathologic features makes determination of the appropriate treatment options challenging. Additional factors such as genomic testing may assist in risk stratification and result in better decision-making.

The FDA has recently approved several new biomarker tests that may help identify which histologically lower-risk cancers may possess higher-risk characteristics. The Oncotype DX prostate biopsy test (Genomic Health, Inc. Redwood City, California) is a multigene assay that evaluates four prostate cancer pathways (androgen signaling, cellular organization, stromal response, and cellular proliferation) to create a Genomic Prostate Score (GPS). The test was validated on biopsy specimens of 431 men with low- and intermediate-risk prostate cancer undergoing radical prostatectomy to determine the association with adverse pathology and recurrence of disease [9]. Adverse pathology was defined as primary Gleason pattern 4 or any pattern 5 and/or pT3 disease. The GPS was significantly associated with adverse pathology with an OR of 2.60 per 20 GPS units. On multivariable analysis, the GPS was the only significant predictor of biochemical recurrence with HR of 2.73 per 20 GPS units. A meta-analysis of 732 patients was conducted to evaluate the ability of GPS to predict pathologic outcomes compared to CAPRA and NCCN risk groups [10]. The study found that the GPS improved the predictive characteristics of both clinical classifiers. The AUC for the NCCN risk groups increased from 0.64 to 0.70, while the AUC for CAPRA increased from 0.68 to 0.73. In a prospective study of 158 patients undergoing treatment for low- or low-intermediate-risk prostate cancer, the GPS was found to be discordant with the NCCN risk in 39% of patients. Further, 18% of patients had changes in treatment recommendation (active surveillance vs. immediate treatment) based on the GPS with an increase in the recommendation of active surveillance from 41 to 51% [11].

The Prolaris test (Myriad Genetics, Salt Lake City, Utah) evaluates a panel of cell cycle progression (CCP) genes to determine the 10-year risk of prostate cancer mortality. The initial study from biopsy-derived tumor tissue included 349 patients who were managed conservatively following cancer diagnosis [12]. On univariate analysis, each unit increase of CCP was associated with a 2.02-fold increase in risk of prostate cancer death. This remained significant even when controlling for biopsy grade and PSA. In a multi-institutional study of 582 men undergoing radical prostatectomy, the CCP score was associated with biochemical recurrence and development of metastatic disease [13]. The CCP score remained a significant predictor of treatment outcomes after controlling for clinical variables. Another recent study of biopsy tissue in patients undergoing radical prostatectomy found mixed results. The CCP score was a significant independent predictor of high-risk prostate cancer, but was not significant for biochemical recurrence after controlling for clinical variables [14].

Moving to broader applicability, the Decipher genomic classifier (GenomeDx, San Diego, California) has been evaluated as a prognostic tool in prostate biopsy tissue. Previously, the test was used following prostatectomy to predict the likelihood of metastases after treatment. However, in a group of 169 men undergoing prostatectomy at Cleveland Clinic, biopsy Decipher was a significant predictor of metastases at 10 years after controlling for clinical variables [15]. The Decipher genomic classifier was also able to predict clinical progression from biopsy tissue in 100 men with intermediate- or high-risk prostate cancer undergoing primary radiation therapy with androgen deprivation therapy [16].

Evaluation

Advances in magnetic resonance imaging (MRI) technology have led to increased imaging for prostate cancer evaluation. Multiparametric MRI (mpMRI), which utilizes several image series, obtains anatomical assessments of the prostate using the T1-weighted (T1W) and T2-weighted (T2W) sequences. The T1W series provides an assessment of hemorrhage that may have occurred on a prior biopsy. The T2W series provides an assessment of structural relationships and details on lesion location. The remaining sequences, diffusion-weighted imaging (DWI) and dynamic contrast-enhanced (DCE) imaging provide assessments of physiologic properties that correlate with prostate cancer detection [17]. The role for prostate imaging with mpMRI has begun to expand. A recent policy statement from the American Urologic Association seeks to address the use of MRI for diagnosis and management of prostate cancer [18]. The decision to obtain a prostate MRI should include an assessment of the quality of imaging available at a particular facility [19]. Variation in image quality and skill of interpretation are known barriers to MRI adoption. It is recommended that all prostate MRI are obtained and reported in accordance with the PI-RADS Version 2 [17, 19].

Patients considering focal therapy will need to undergo imaging to determine the size and location of the lesion that will be treated. Focal therapy is based on the principle that treatment of an index lesion will provide meaningful cancer control without the detrimental side effects from treating the reminder of the prostate [20]. The index lesion is typically defined as the largest or highest-grade lesion. In a study of patients undergoing prostatectomy, Russo et al. have shown that mpMRI is highly sensitive for detecting the index lesion [21]. For patients undergoing prostate biopsy, mpMRI can be used to biopsy the index lesion. In a retrospective study of 135 patients undergoing prostatectomy, the index lesion identified on MRI-transrectal ultrasound (TRUS) fusion biopsy was concordant with prostatectomy pathology in 95% of patients [22].

Prostate cancer detection for patients considering enrollment in an active surveillance program is important to ensure that no clinically significant cancer is missed and to ensure that any potential disease progression would not preclude definitive local therapy options. Patients already on an active surveillance protocol may elect to obtain a mpMRI in place of repeated biopsy. However, the data supporting sequential prostate MRI as part of an active surveillance program is lacking [23]. In a study of patients on active surveillance who underwent serial mpMRI and subsequent biopsy, the sensitivity and specificity for mpMRI to detect a change in Gleason score were 53% and 80%, respectively [24]. To improve our understanding of prostate MRI for men on active surveillance, a European School of Oncology Task Force recently released the PRECISE recommendations for collecting data on MRIs obtained during active surveillance [25]. The lack of data and the potential that an MRI may miss clinically significant cancer that would be detected on repeat biopsy has led to the recommendation that imaging alone cannot be the sole means of monitoring men on active surveillance [18].

The confirmatory biopsy is a part of most active surveillance protocols and represents the first planned biopsy after diagnosis with prostate cancer. It can also be incorporated into treatment planning for focal therapy. For the purposes of active surveillance, the repeat biopsy serves to overcome limitations in cancer detection from under sampling. Reports from early active surveillance cohorts found that 20–30% of patients were no longer candidates for surveillance following confirmatory biopsy [26]. Attempts to improve detection of clinically significant prostate cancer have relied on incorporation of mpMRI into confirmatory biopsy protocols. Improved prostate cancer detection can also overcome limitations that resulted in the advocacy of extended template biopsies and saturation biopsies. In a study of 41 low-risk patients undergoing confirmatory biopsy using systematic biopsy and MRI-targeted biopsies, 59% of patients were reclassified. The MRI-targeted biopsy was responsible for reclassification in 20% of patients [27]. In another study of 105 patients undergoing confirmatory biopsy with mpMRI, 60% of patients had highly suspicious lesions on MRI (PI-RADS 4–5). The systematic biopsy identified significant cancer in 45% of patients. Targeting lesions found on MRI identified an additional 10 cases, raising the detection of significant cancer to 56% [28].

Technological advances have resulted in fusion of the MRI images with real-time TRUS images to guide prostate biopsies. For men undergoing a confirmatory biopsy or in those who may undergo repeat biopsy prior to focal therapy, fusion biopsy offers potential improvements in prostate cancer detection. In a study of 207 men undergoing fusion biopsy as a part of active surveillance, Tran et al. found that 83 men (40%) were upgraded [29]. The systematic biopsy resulted in upgrading in 49 (24%) patients, while the targeted biopsy identified significant cancer in 30 (14%) patients. Two patients had significant cancer found on both biopsies. In a similar study of 54 patients undergoing confirmatory biopsy using MRI-US fusion-directed biopsies, significant cancer was found in 12 patients (22%) [30]. The addition of targeted biopsies increased significant cancer detection from 17% on systematic biopsy alone. The sensitivity for detecting significant cancer was higher for systematic biopsies than for targeted biopsies. In both studies, the importance of performing a concomitant systematic biopsy is supported.

Saturation biopsy has been proposed as a gold standard for prostate cancer detection. Early studies found that transperineal saturation mapping biopsies could be used to identify clinically significant cancer and plan for focal therapy [31]. The advances in mpMRI had created hope that MRI-US fusion biopsies would provide comparable detection of clinically significant prostate cancer without the need for saturation biopsy. In a small study of 40 men on active surveillance, Pepe et al. compared the results of transperineal saturation biopsy (median 30 cores) with fusion guided TRUS biopsy of PR-RADS 3–4 lesions (median 4 cores) [32]. Of the patients, ten were reclassified based on results from the saturation biopsy. The authors found that mpMRI detected all of the potentially clinically significant lesions. However, fusion biopsy failed to identify 3/10 significant prostate cancers. This study was limited by the lack of systematic biopsies in combination with targeted biopsies.

Larger studies of patients undergoing fusion-guided biopsy of targeted lesion have found better detection of clinically significant cancer. Radtke et al. set out to study 294 consecutive men undergoing combined transperineal template saturation biopsy and MRI-guided targeted biopsy [33]. The group included 108 patients undergoing repeat biopsy. Combined, the systematic and targeted biopsies detected 86 clinically significant cancers. However, the systematic missed 18 (20.9%) significant tumors, while the targeted biopsy missed 11 (12.8%). The targeted biopsies were successful in missing 43.8% of Gleason 6 tumors. However, limiting the biopsy to only PI-RADS 3–5 lesions would have resulted in missing 17 significant cancers. The results support a combined systematic and targeted biopsy as the gold standard for prostate cancer detection. The PROMIS study was a large multicenter study evaluating the role of mpMRI in primary prostate biopsy using image-directed biopsy compared to transperineal template prostate mapping biopsy [34]. The study included over 500 men who underwent mpMRI followed by mapping biopsy and TRUS biopsy. The study found that including mpMRI prior to biopsy would improve the detection of clinically significant prostate cancer by 18% while potentially reducing the detection of clinically insignificant cancer by 5%. Following this study, the NCCN guidelines updated the prostate cancer early detection indication for biopsy to include the consideration of mpMRI prior to prostate biopsy.

Therapeutic Management

Active Surveillance

Active surveillance is based on a regimen of serial evaluations over time to ensure that sampling error or disease progression is identified early, allowing for definitive treatment. However, several different active surveillance protocols are described, and there is wide variation in the implementation among different providers. In a survey of nearly 400 urologists who manage patients on active surveillance, Gorin et al. found a wide variation in criteria for enrollment and management while on active surveillance [35]. More than half (58%) of those surveyed reported obtaining a confirmatory biopsy at the 12-month mark; however, 30% preferred to obtain the biopsy earlier, between 1 and 9 months. Only 24% of respondents felt that MRI played a role in active surveillance monitoring.

Several large prospective studies have reported outcomes from differing active surveillance protocols and can be used as a reference point for creating a follow-up regimen. The Johns Hopkins protocol includes a confirmatory biopsy within 12 months of initiation, along with PSA and DRE every 6 months [36]. Uniquely, the protocol recommends a follow-up biopsy every 12 months to ensure high-grade cancers are not missed. The authors suggest that with improvements in imaging and genomic testing, a less rigorous biopsy schedule may achieve the same results. The Toronto cohort represents a similarly robust program of active surveillance with a less aggressive biopsy regimen [37]. Although the confirmatory biopsy is obtained within 12 months of enrollment, subsequent biopsies are spaced out up to 3–4 years. Serial PSA testing occurs every 3 months for the first 2 years and then becomes biannual going forward. The Canary Prostate Active Surveillance Study (PASS) represents yet another well-studied active surveillance regimen [38]. Men in this study undergo quarterly PSA testing, biannual DRE, a confirmatory biopsy within 6–12 months of enrollment, and serial biopsies every 2 years thereafter.

For patients undergoing active surveillance, it is important to recognize that although they are not receiving active treatment, they may still notice changes in sexual and urinary symptoms secondary to the diagnosis of cancer and required evaluations [39]. In a large, prospective quality of life study of men undergoing local treatment for prostate cancer or watchful waiting, early urinary leakage and sexual function scores were more favorable in the watchful waiting group [40]. However, with longer follow-up, men in the watchful waiting group experienced a significant reduction in quality of life that was not seen in the prostatectomy group [41]. A separate study using the CaPSURE database to compare mental health and quality of life in patients undergoing prostatectomy, radiation therapy, or watchful waiting also found treatment-associated differences in quality of life [42]. Reported mental health domains were initially similar; however, with long-term follow-up, patients undergoing prostatectomy reported significantly better mental health quality, followed by patients on watchful waiting and finally patients undergoing radiation therapy. The potential avoidance of early sexual and urinary health side effects may be balanced by changes in quality of mental health, although the approach to watchful waiting is likely less rigorous than undergoing active surveillance.

The reliance on repetitive biopsies during active surveillance has been proposed as one potential cause of sexual health deterioration. In a study from Johns Hopkins of 333 men undergoing active surveillance, biopsy number was associated with a decrease in scores for the Sexual Health Inventory for Men (SHIM) [43]. For men who have undergone three or more biopsies, a significantly greater reduction was noted than for those with two or fewer biopsies. Interestingly, the number of biopsies was not correlated with changes in lower urinary tract symptoms. The group from UCSF reported on their cohort of 427 men undergoing active surveillance [44]. Using the SHIM, they separately evaluated sexual function and sexual activity. They did not find a significant association with erectile function scores and biopsy number. Although results differ regarding the impact of serial biopsies on erectile function, it should be noted that any sexual health decline caused by prostate biopsy is likely to be much less in magnitude than that which would occur from definitive local therapy.

Focal Therapy

Focal therapy represents a novel treatment strategy using a heterogeneous group of energy sources that aims to destroy prostate tissue in a controlled fashion without removal or treatment of the entire prostate. By localizing treatment, surrounding vital structures including the rectum, bladder neck, and neurovascular bundles are spared by the effects of treatment. Several energy sources have been evaluated for effectiveness in focal therapy. The two most widely studied treatment modalities are high-intensity focused ultrasound (HIFU) and cryotherapy. However, other devices including irreversible electroporation, photodynamic therapy, and interstitial laser have been proposed as tools for focal therapy [45].

Cryotherapy is a thermally ablative treatment that relies on rapid reduction of prostate gland temperature followed by tissue warming to cause microvascular injury, cell wall disruption, and eventually cell death. Ice ball formation during cryotherapy is achieved using treatment probes placed in a transperineal position. Therapy is monitored using ultrasound to follow ice propagation and ensure vital structures are not injured. Several studies have reported outcomes on cryotherapy. The national Cryo On-Line Database (COLD) registry was created to facilitate systematic investigations of cryotherapy outcomes. In a review of patients included in the COLD Registry from 1997 to 2007, Ward et al. identified 1160 patients (19.8%) undergoing focal therapy [5]. They evaluated for oncologic and functional outcomes. Using ASTRO definition for biochemical recurrence, they found that at 2 years, 75.7% of patients were free from recurrence. Prostate biopsy was obtained in only 164 patients (14.1%) with 43 patients having residual cancer (26.3%). Functional outcomes were also evaluated. Urinary continence, defined as freedom from pads, was achieved in 98.4%. New-onset erectile dysfunction was reported in 41.9% of patients. In summary, this study of cryotherapy functional and oncologic outcomes from a group that infrequently performed posttreatment biopsy found few recurrences with minimal urinary symptoms but appreciable declines in erectile function.

HIFU is a focal therapy approach that causes prostate tissue ablation by both thermal and mechanical disruption. High-intensity ultrasound waves pass from a transducer in the rectum into the prostate focusing on a small area, resulting in cavitation and coagulative necrosis [45]. Treatment is monitored simultaneously using live ultrasound and temperature monitoring. Several studies have reported on the outcomes of a limited number of patients; however, there are no randomized studies to compare outcomes between HIFU and other established treatments. In a systematic review of patients undergoing HIFU therapy, Golan et al. found a wide variation in patient selection, treatment strategy, and post-ablation follow-up [46]. From 13 studies of patients undergoing focal HIFU, they identified 11 primary focal therapy studies comprising 456 patients. Of these patients, 103 had a positive posttreatment biopsy with 30 (8%) having clinically significant disease. Ultimately 44 patients (10%) underwent additional therapy with either repeat HIFU, prostatectomy, radiation therapy, or hormonal ablation. In a separate systematic review of 346 patients undergoing focal HIFU, Valerio et al. reported that prostate cancer was detected in 23.3% of patients undergoing posttreatment biopsy [45]. In the systematic reviews of HIFU treatment, functional outcomes varied widely between studies. However, in a pooled analysis, incontinence was reported in only 3.7% of patients with no patients requiring pads. Intact erectile function was reported in 88.6% of patients with 13.8% requiring new PDE-5 inhibitor usage following treatment [45]. A recent prospective study of 54 men undergoing focal therapy with HIFU found a drop in the mean PSA from 6.2 to 2.9 at the 12-month visit [47]. Similar to outcomes in the systematic reviews, residual cancer was detected in 26.5% of patients at the 12-month biopsy with 8.2% having persistent clinically significant cancer. Salvage treatment was undertaken by 19.6% of patients. Incontinence developed in 3.9% of patients after treatment. Erectile function was maintained in 70% of patients that were potent prior to focal therapy.

Emerging technologies may ultimately provide improvements over HIFU or cryotherapy for focal treatment of localized prostate cancer. Irreversible electroporation has been proposed as a treatment that can locally ablate prostate tissue by disruption of cellular membranes following repetitive electrical pulses. In a small study of 63 patients undergoing focal therapy with irreversible electroporation, 70% of patients experienced a PSA decline at 6–12 months, and 76% were free of cancer on follow-up biopsy [48]. However, use of irreversible electroporation is made difficult by the lack of treatment monitoring. Further, treatment can be halted by system errors based on the delivery of current, which occurred in seven patients from this study and was associated with in-field disease on re-biopsy.

Lasers have also been employed to focally ablate prostate cancer tissue. Focal laser ablation relies on direct thermal injury from laser excitation within the area of treatment. Several small studies have provided data on a select group of patients [45]. Additional studies will be required to determine the oncologic and functional results following laser therapy. Photodynamic therapy is another focal treatment that utilizes laser energy; however, laser excitation results in activation of a vascular photosensitizer which causes vascular damage and cell death. Recently a phase 3 randomized trial of photodynamic therapy versus active surveillance for patients with low-risk prostate cancer was published [49]. The co-primary end points were treatment failure and absence of definitive cancer at 24 months. The study included 414 patients. At 24 months, disease progression occurred in 28% of photodynamic patients and 58% of active surveillance patients. A negative biopsy was found in 49% of photodynamic patients but only 14% of active surveillance patients. The authors concluded that photodynamic therapy is safe and effective for patients with low-risk prostate cancer.

Beyond the technical challenges of focally treating prostate cancer, the follow-up of patients undergoing focal therapy is complicated by the presence of residual healthy prostate tissue. Potential follow-up options include digital rectal exam, PSA measurement, mpMRI studies, and serial prostate biopsies. However, interpretations of results from PSA and MRI reflect the presence of treated lesions and adjacent normal tissue. New definitions of treatment success and failure are required. Focal treatment failure can be described as persistence of cancer in a treated area [50]. This requires image-guided re-biopsy of previously treated areas. Conversely, prostate cancer recurrence could be defined as rising PSA following treatment or detection of prostate cancer outside the focally treated area. The lack of discrimination between treatment failure and recurrence makes interpretation of focal therapy studies difficult.

Following prostatectomy, PSA is used to confirm treatment success and monitor for recurrence. Because residual healthy tissue continues to make PSA, and reductions in PSA may not be as significant as with whole gland therapy, follow-up PSA must be interpreted carefully. Many studies have relied on definitions derived from prostate radiotherapy, including the Phoenix and ASTRO criteria. However, there is not a clear relationship between PSA kinetics and treatment failure in patients undergoing focal therapy, and use of radiotherapy definitions may not reflect treatment outcomes. Because the index lesion is felt to be a major contributor to the PSA level, a reduction in PSA of 50% has been proposed as a target within 3 months of treatment. Regardless of PSA reductions, the stability of the posttreatment PSA represents an important indicator of treatment success [50].

Focal therapy is predicated on detection of lesions within the prostate using imaging such as MRI. Continued serial imaging is needed to monitor patients following focal therapy and allows correlation of PSA with treatment effects on gland size while also imaging the contralateral untreated tissue. Posttreatment MRI images may vary by energy source, but generally areas of treatment will display altered structural appearance with loss of enhancement, scarring, and fibrosis. Follow-up MRI studies are also useful for conducting posttreatment biopsies of both the treatment zone and the remaining untreated prostate tissue as part of continued surveillance. Dickinson et al. conducted a pooled analysis of three HIFU studies to evaluate the accuracy of follow-up prostate MRI and PSA measurements for predicting residual cancer following focal therapy [51]. They identified 111 men who underwent serial PSA evaluations, prostate MRI, and biopsy 6 months following treatment. They found residual prostate cancer in 25% of patients with clinically significant disease in 12 patients. MRI at 6 months was more accurate for predicting residual prostate cancer than any PSA measurements including PSA nadir and PSA density.

Following focal therapy, patients who are found to have treatment failure or disease progression are often recommended salvage therapy. As with salvage treatment after failed radiation therapy, there is concern for worse oncologic and functional outcomes with post-focal salvage therapies. To evaluate the results of salvage prostatectomy following focal therapy, Nunes-Silva et al. evaluated 22 men in a matched cohort study of patients undergoing prostatectomy [52]. They found similar complication and pad-free rates. However, recovery of erectile function was significantly worse in the patients undergoing salvage prostatectomy and corresponded to fewer patients receiving nerve sparing in the salvage setting. They also found that the risk of biochemical recurrence was significantly higher in patients who received salvage prostatectomy. Salvage treatment following focal therapy is feasible and safe but may result in worse sexual function and higher chances of disease recurrence compared to upfront prostatectomy.

Given the challenges of detecting focal therapy failure with recurrence or progression, close follow-up of patients is required. There is no specific follow-up regimen that has been proven superior. However, several common recommendations have been provided. In a consensus project of focal therapy experts, Muller et al. recommend using PSA, mpMRI, fusion biopsies, and quality of life measures to follow patients after focal therapy [53]. For the first year, PSA measurements should be obtained every 3 months, then every 6 months going beyond. Prostate MRI is recommended at 6 months as a baseline, then at 12 months, and annually thereafter. A follow-up biopsy should be obtained at 12 months, ideally using MRI fusion. The biopsy should include 4–6 cores from the treatment zone in addition to a 12-core systematic biopsy. A similar expert consensus report also recommends a 12-month follow-up biopsy to ensure adequate treatment [54].

Conclusions

Active surveillance has been proposed as a way to continue current prostate cancer screening programs while mitigating the risk of prostate cancer overdetection. Conversely, focal therapy has often been criticized based on the potential that multifocal disease may be missed. Unfortunately, the development of clinical trials to evaluate focal treatment of prostate cancer has been hampered by the uncertainty with end points, the need for very long follow-up, and the desires by patients to undergo novel treatments in hopes that side effects will be minimized [55].

In this clinical scenario, a 58-year-old man with a normal rectal exam presents with a PSA that is below the typical threshold but may be considered elevated after adjustment for age. He has undergone a systematic transrectal ultrasound-guided biopsy with low-intermediate-risk prostate cancer identified in 1 out of 12 cores. He is now considering active surveillance or focal therapy.

Any patient considering focal therapy should undergo prostate imaging with a mpMRI to determine their candidacy for this treatment. This MRI should be appropriately spaced to ensure the best possible imaging with minimal distortion from the preceding biopsy. For patients who have no index lesion identified, additional evaluation with genomic testing may improve risk stratification or exclude active surveillance as an option. After the MRI, patients who remain interested in focal therapy may desire a biopsy to confirm that the lesion is actually intermediate-risk and not higher-grade disease. Many patients who present as intermediate risk are found to be higher risk on subsequent biopsy with appropriate targeting of the index lesion. The location of the index lesion may factor in deciding which treatment modality would be best suited for focal therapy. Patient and provider should consider all options and discuss the risk and benefits of each.

This patient elected to proceed with mpMRI of the prostate. The T2-weighted images are found in Fig. 5.1. A single index lesion was identified, and subsequent MRI/ultrasound fusion biopsy confirmed the presence of intermediate-risk disease. After considering the options, the patient elected focal cryotherapy of the index lesion. The patient had a follow-up MRI and fusion biopsy that confirmed successful treatment.

For any patient considering focal therapy, starting the discussion with active surveillance (i.e., keeping an intact prostate) sets the stage for discussions of partial gland treatment. The risks for cancer progression following focal therapy

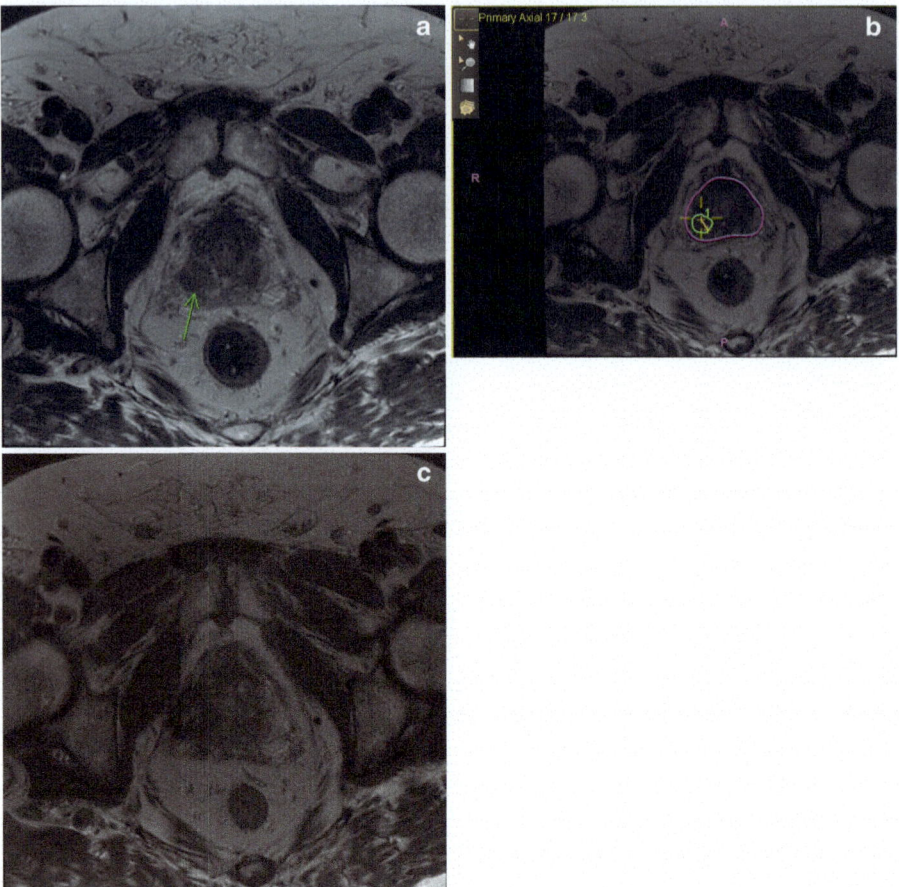

Fig. 5.1 Focal cryotherapy of intermediate-risk prostate cancer. A single index lesion was identified with low-intermediate-risk prostate cancer on fusion biopsy. (**a**) T2-weighted MRI of the prostate showing a PI-RADS 4 lesion in the right peripheral zone. (**b**) MRI/US fusion-guided prostate biopsy. (**c**) Posttreatment T2-weighted MRI of the prostate showing scarring of the ablation site without evidence of persistent disease, confirmed with biopsy

should be no worse than those on active surveillance and no better than those undergoing prostatectomy. As diagnostic precision increases, the management of prostate cancer can begin to take on a continuum of invasiveness from active surveillance, to focal therapy, to whole gland treatment (Fig. 5.2). The future will likely be shaped by current studies of novel targeted treatments for men who are on active surveillance. Promising results from these early studies seem to indicate that a new progressive treatment paradigm for managing prostate cancer may be on the horizon [49].

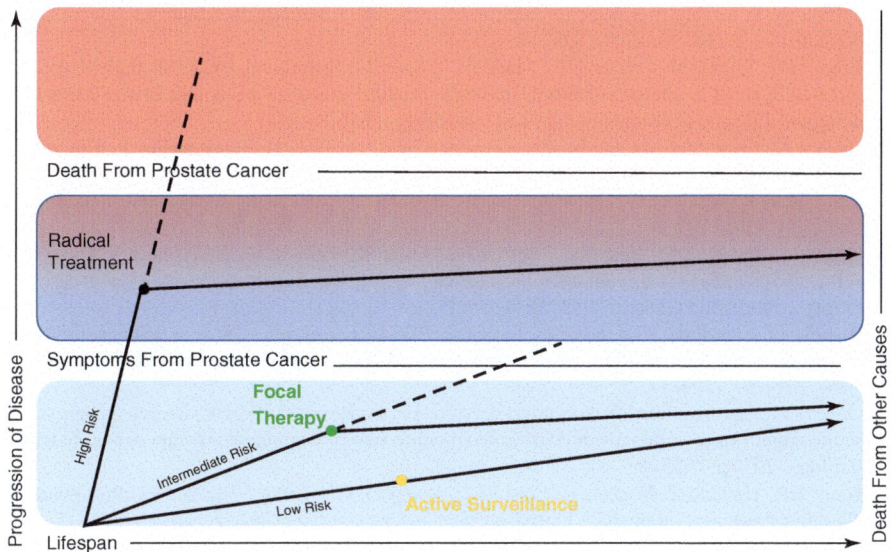

Fig. 5.2 Risk-stratified treatment of prostate cancer in the era of focal therapy and active surveillance. Prostate cancer treatment is intended to prevent death or debilitating symptoms from prostate cancer progression. Men with high-risk prostate cancer should undergo definitive therapy. Those with low risk should be eligible for active surveillance. Focal therapy may represent a treatment option best suited for men with intermediate-risk prostate cancer

References

1. Sakr WA, Grignon DJ, Crissman JD, Heilbrun LK, Cassin BJ, Pontes JJ, et al. High grade prostatic intraepithelial neoplasia (HGPIN) and prostatic adenocarcinoma between the ages of 20-69: an autopsy study of 249 cases. In Vivo. 1994;8:439–43.
2. Siegel RL, Miller KD, Jemal A. Cancer statistics, 2017. CA Cancer J Clin. 2017;67:7–30.
3. D'Amico AV, Whittington R, Malkowicz SB, Schultz D, Blank K, Broderick GA, et al. Biochemical outcome after radical prostatectomy, external beam radiation therapy, or interstitial radiation therapy for clinically localized prostate cancer. JAMA. 1998;280:969–74.
4. Morlacco A, Cheville JC, Rangel LJ, Gearman DJ, Karnes RJ. Adverse disease features in Gleason score 3 + 4 "favorable intermediate-risk" prostate cancer: implications for active surveillance. Eur Urol. 2017;72:442–7.
5. Ward JF, Jones JS. Focal cryotherapy for localized prostate cancer: a report from the national Cryo On-Line Database (COLD) registry. BJU Int. 2012;109:1648–54.
6. Ahmed HU, Arya M, Freeman A, Emberton M. Do low-grade and low-volume prostate cancers bear the hallmarks of malignancy? Lancet Oncol. 2012;13:e509–17.
7. Ross HM, Kryvenko ON, Cowan JE, Simko JP, Wheeler TM, Epstein JI. Do adenocarcinomas of the prostate with Gleason score (GS)≤6 have the potential to metastasize to lymph nodes? Am J Surg Pathol. 2012;36:1346–52.
8. Dinh KT, Mahal BA, Ziehr DR, Muralidhar V, Chen Y-W, Viswanathan VB, et al. Incidence and predictors of upgrading and up staging among 10,000 contemporary patients with low risk prostate cancer. J Urol. 2015;194:343–9.
9. Cullen J, Rosner IL, Brand TC, Zhang N, Tsiatis AC, Moncur J, et al. A biopsy-based 17-gene genomic prostate score predicts recurrence after radical prostatectomy and adverse surgical

pathology in a racially diverse population of men with clinically low- and intermediate-risk prostate cancer. Eur Urol. 2015;68:123–31.

10. Brand TC, Zhang N, Crager MR, Maddala T, Dee A, Sesterhenn IA, et al. Patient-specific meta-analysis of 2 clinical validation studies to predict pathologic outcomes in prostate cancer using the 17-gene genomic prostate score. Urology. 2016;89:69–75.

11. Badani KK, Kemeter MJ, Febbo PG, Lawrence HJ, Denes BS, Rothney MP, et al. The impact of a biopsy based 17-gene genomic prostate score on treatment recommendations in men with newly diagnosed clinically prostate cancer who are candidates for active surveillance. Urol Pract. 2015;2:181–9.

12. Cuzick J, Berney DM, Fisher G, Mesher D, Møller H, Reid JE, et al. Prognostic value of a cell cycle progression signature for prostate cancer death in a conservatively managed needle biopsy cohort. Br J Cancer. 2012;106:1095–9.

13. Bishoff JT, Freedland SJ, Gerber L, Tennstedt P, Reid J, Welbourn W, et al. Prognostic utility of the cell cycle progression score generated from biopsy in men treated with prostatectomy. J Urol. 2014;192:409–14.

14. Oderda M, Cozzi G, Daniele L, Sapino A, Munegato S, Renne G, et al. Cell-cycle progression-score might improve the current risk assessment in newly diagnosed prostate cancer patients. Urology. 2017;102:73–8.

15. Klein EA, Haddad Z, Yousefi K, Lam LLC, Wang Q, Choeurng V, et al. Decipher genomic classifier measured on prostate biopsy predicts metastasis risk. Urology. 2016;90:148–52.

16. Nguyen PL, Martin NE, Choeurng V, Palmer-Aronsten B, Kolisnik T, Beard CJ, et al. Utilization of biopsy-based genomic classifier to predict distant metastasis after definitive radiation and short-course ADT for intermediate and high-risk prostate cancer. Prostate Cancer Prostatic Dis. 2017;20:186–92.

17. Weinreb JC, Barentsz JO, Choyke PL, Cornud F, Haider MA, Macura KJ, et al. PI-RADS prostate imaging—reporting and data system: 2015, version 2. Eur Urol. 2016;69:16–40.

18. Fulgham PF, Rukstalis DB, Turkbey IB, Rubenstein JN, Taneja S, Carroll PR, et al. AUA policy statement on the use of multiparametric magnetic resonance imaging in the diagnosis, staging and management of prostate cancer. J Urol. 2017;198:832–8.

19. Rosenkrantz AB, Verma S, Choyke P, Eberhardt SC, Eggener SE, Gaitonde K, et al. Prostate magnetic resonance imaging and magnetic resonance imaging targeted biopsy in patients with a prior negative biopsy: a consensus statement by AUA and SAR. J Urol. 2016;196:1613–8.

20. Ahmed HU. The index lesion and the origin of prostate cancer. N Engl J Med. 2009;361:1704–6.

21. Russo F, Regge D, Armando E, Giannini V, Vignati A, Mazzetti S, et al. Detection of prostate cancer index lesions with multiparametric magnetic resonance imaging (mp-MRI) using whole-mount histological sections as the reference standard. BJU Int. 2016;118(1):84–94.

22. Baco E, Ukimura O, Rud E, Vlatkovic L, Svindland A, Aron M, et al. Magnetic resonance imaging-transectal ultrasound image-fusion biopsies accurately characterize the index tumor: correlation with step-sectioned radical prostatectomy specimens in 135 patients. Eur Urol. 2015;67(4):787–94. https://doi.org/10.1016/j.eururo.2014.08.077.

23. Schoots IG, Petrides N, Giganti F, Bokhorst LP, Rannikko A, Klotz L, et al. Magnetic resonance imaging in active surveillance of prostate cancer: a systematic review. Eur Urol. 2015;67:627–36.

24. Walton-Diaz A, Shakir NA, George AK, Rais-Bahrami S, Turkbey B, Rothwax JT, et al. Use of serial multiparametric magnetic resonance imaging in the management of patients with prostate cancer on active surveillance. Urol Oncol. 2015;33:202.e1–7.

25. Moore CM, Giganti F, Albertsen P, Allen C, Bangma C, Briganti A, et al. Reporting magnetic resonance imaging in men on active surveillance for prostate cancer: the PRECISE recommendations-a report of a European School of Oncology task force. Eur Urol. 2017;71:648–55.

26. Dall'Era MA, Albertsen PC, Bangma C, Carroll PR, Carter HB, Cooperberg MR, et al. Active surveillance for prostate cancer: a systematic review of the literature. Eur Urol. 2012;62:976–83.

27. Marliere F, Puech P, Benkirane A, Villers A, Lemaitre L, Leroy X, et al. The role of MRI-targeted and confirmatory biopsies for cancer upstaging at selection in patients considered for active surveillance for clinically low-risk prostate cancer. World J Urol. 2014;32:951–8.
28. Pessoa RR, Viana PC, Mattedi RL, Guglielmetti GB, Cordeiro MD, Coelho RF, et al. Value of 3-tesla multiparametric magnetic resonance imaging and targeted biopsy for improved risk stratification in patients considered for active surveillance. BJU Int. 2017;119:535–42.
29. Tran GN, Leapman MS, Nguyen HG, Cowan JE, Shinohara K, Westphalen AC, et al. Magnetic resonance imaging-ultrasound fusion biopsy during prostate cancer active surveillance. Eur Urol. 2017;72:275–81.
30. Ma TM, Tosoian JJ, Schaeffer EM, Landis P, Wolf S, Macura KJ, et al. The role of multiparametric magnetic resonance imaging/ultrasound fusion biopsy in active surveillance. Eur Urol. 2017;71:174–80.
31. Barzell WE, Melamed MR. Appropriate patient selection in the focal treatment of prostate cancer: the role of transperineal 3-dimensional pathologic mapping of the prostate—a 4-year experience. Urology. 2007;70:27–35.
32. Pepe P, Garufi A, Priolo G, Pennisi M. Can MRI/TRUS fusion targeted biopsy replace saturation prostate biopsy in the re-evaluation of men in active surveillance? World J Urol. 2016;34:1249–53.
33. Radtke JP, Kuru TH, Boxler S, Alt CD, Popeneciu IV, Huettenbrink C, et al. Comparative analysis of transperineal template saturation prostate biopsy versus magnetic resonance imaging targeted biopsy with magnetic resonance imaging-ultrasound fusion guidance. J Urol. 2015;193:87–94.
34. Ahmed HU, El-Shater Bosaily A, Brown LC, Gabe R, Kaplan R, Parmar MK, et al. Diagnostic accuracy of multi-parametric MRI and TRUS biopsy in prostate cancer (PROMIS): a paired validating confirmatory study. Lancet. 2017;389:815–22.
35. Gorin MA, Eldefrawy A, Ekwenna O, Soloway MS. Active surveillance for low-risk prostate cancer: knowledge, acceptance and practice among urologists. Prostate Cancer Prostatic Dis. 2012;15:177–81.
36. Tosoian JJ, Mamawala M, Epstein JI, Landis P, Wolf S, Trock BJ, et al. Intermediate and longer-term outcomes from a prospective active-surveillance program for favorable-risk prostate cancer. J Clin Oncol. 2015;33:3379–85.
37. Klotz L, Vesprini D, Sethukavalan P, Jethava V, Zhang L, Jain S, et al. Long-term follow-up of a large active surveillance cohort of patients with prostate cancer. J Clin Oncol. 2015;33:272–7.
38. Newcomb LF, Brooks JD, Carroll PR, Feng Z, Gleave ME, Nelson PS, et al. Canary prostate active surveillance study: design of a multi-institutional active surveillance cohort and biorepository. Urology. 2010;75:407–13.
39. Bergman J, Litwin MS. Quality of life in men undergoing active surveillance for localized prostate cancer. J Natl Cancer Inst Monogr. 2012;2012:242–9.
40. Steineck G, Helgesen F, Adolfsson J, Dickman PW, Johansson J-E, Norlén BJ, et al. Quality of life after radical prostatectomy or watchful waiting. N Engl J Med. 2002;347:790–6.
41. Johansson E, Bill-Axelson A, Holmberg L, Onelöv E, Johansson J-E, Steineck G, et al. Time, symptom burden, androgen deprivation, and self-assessed quality of life after radical prostatectomy or watchful waiting: the Randomized Scandinavian Prostate Cancer Group Study Number 4 (SPCG-4) clinical trial. Eur Urol. 2009;55:422–30.
42. Litwin MS, Lubeck DP, Spitalny GM, Henning JM, Carroll PR. Mental health in men treated for early stage prostate carcinoma: a posttreatment, longitudinal quality of life analysis from the Cancer of the Prostate Strategic Urologic Research Endeavor. Cancer. 2002;95:54–60.
43. Fujita K, Landis P, McNeil BK, Pavlovich CP. Serial prostate biopsies are associated with an increased risk of erectile dysfunction in men with prostate cancer on active surveillance. J Urol. 2009;182:2664–9.
44. Hilton JF, Blaschko SD, Whitson JM, Cowan JE, Carroll PR. The impact of serial prostate biopsies on sexual function in men on active surveillance for prostate cancer. J Urol. 2012;188:1252–8.

45. Valerio M, Cerantola Y, Eggener SE, Lepor H, Polascik TJ, Villers A, et al. New and established technology in focal ablation of the prostate: a systematic review. Eur Urol. 2017;71:17–34.
46. Golan R, Bernstein AN, McClure TD, Sedrakyan A, Patel NA, Parekh DJ, et al. Partial gland treatment of prostate cancer using high-intensity focused ultrasound in the primary and salvage settings: a systematic review. J Urol. 2017;198:1000–9.
47. Ganzer R, Hadaschik B, Pahernik S, Koch D, Baumunk D, Kuru T, et al. Prospective multicenter phase II-study on focal therapy (hemiablation) of the prostate with high intensity focused ultrasound (HIFU). J Urol. 2017. https://doi.org/10.1016/j.juro.2017.10.033.
48. van den Bos W, Scheltema MJ, Siriwardana AR, Kalsbeek AMF, Thompson JE, Ting F, et al. Focal irreversible electroporation as primary treatment for localized prostate cancer. BJU Int. 2017. https://doi.org/10.1111/bju.13983.
49. Azzouzi A-R, Vincendeau S, Barret E, Cicco A, Kleinclauss F, van der Poel HG, et al. Padeliporfin vascular-targeted photodynamic therapy versus active surveillance in men with low-risk prostate cancer (CLIN1001 PCM301): an open-label, phase 3, randomised controlled trial. Lancet Oncol. 2017;18:181–91.
50. Barret E, Harvey-Bryan K-A, Sanchez-Salas R, Rozet F, Galiano M, Cathelineau X. How to diagnose and treat focal therapy failure and recurrence? Curr Opin Urol. 2014;24:241–6.
51. Dickinson L, Ahmed HU, Hindley RG, McCartan N, Freeman A, Allen C, et al. Prostate-specific antigen vs. magnetic resonance imaging parameters for assessing oncological outcomes after high intensity-focused ultrasound focal therapy for localized prostate cancer. Urol Oncol. 2017;35:30.e9–30.e15.
52. Nunes-Silva I, Barret E, Srougi V, Baghdadi M, Capogrosso P, Garcia-Barreras S, et al. Effect of prior focal therapy on perioperative, oncologic and functional outcomes of salvage robotic assisted radical prostatectomy. J Urol. 2017;198:1069–76.
53. Muller BG, Van den Bos W, Brausi M, Fütterer JJ, Ghai S, Pinto PA, et al. Follow-up modalities in focal therapy for prostate cancer: results from a Delphi consensus project. World J Urol. 2015;33:1503–9.
54. Donaldson IA, Alonzi R, Barratt D, Barret E, Berge V, Bott S, et al. Focal therapy: patients, interventions, and outcomes--a report from a consensus meeting. Eur Urol. 2015;67(4):771–7.
55. Jarow JP, Thompson IM, Kluetz PG, Baxley J, Sridhara R, Scardino P, et al. Drug and device development for localized prostate cancer: report of a Food and Drug Administration/American Urological Association public workshop. Urology. 2014;83(5):975–8.

Chapter 6
Prostate Cancer Treatment Options for Men with Significant Urinary Symptoms and Enlarged Prostates

Cary N. Robertson

Clinical Case Scenario: A 74-year-old man with Gleason 7 (3 + 4) prostate cancer with significant lower urinary tract symptoms (LUTS) and AUA symptom score 21 declines radical prostatectomy.

Radiation therapy or an ablative technique such as cryotherapy or high-intensity focused ultrasound (HIFU) may provide effective cancer treatment. These treatments, however, present a risk of urinary retention, urinary incontinence, urethral stricture, and bladder neck contracture, especially in enlarged, symptomatic prostates [1, 2]. Prostate size reduction may reduce these risks and can be accomplished by hormonal downsizing or minimally invasive endosurgical techniques [3–5]. Such a tissue reduction strategy alleviates bladder obstruction, preserves bladder function, and reduces the risk of urinary retention post-therapy. Endosurgical resection or enucleation of obstructing glandular tissue may be more effective than hormonal downsizing. Both techniques may be used in combination for maximum effect. Prostate cancer therapy combined with prostate size reduction is an optimal approach in this case example.

Evaluation

The evaluation of prostate size and symptoms determines treatment choice in certain patients. While definitive therapy choices include surgery, radiation therapy, and ablative approaches such as cryotherapy and HIFU, this patient does not desire

C. N. Robertson, M.D., F.A.C.S. (✉)
Division of Urology, Department of Surgery,
Duke University Medical Center, Durham, NC, USA
e-mail: cary.robertson@duke.edu

© Springer International Publishing AG, part of Springer Nature 2018   75
S. S. Chang, M. S. Cookson (eds.), *Prostate Cancer*,
https://doi.org/10.1007/978-3-319-78646-9_6

radical surgery. In addition, the prostate measures 60 cm^3 with significant lower urinary tract symptoms (LUTS) and an American Urological Association (AUA) symptom score of 21 out of 35. This complicates his management. It may be presumed that he has urinary tract obstruction. He is at risk for exacerbation of symptoms posttreatment. Prostate gland size reduction via hormonal therapy or endosurgical techniques may be needed. Prior to such measures, however, confirmatory urodynamic testing is frequently helpful. At a minimum, bladder scan and flow rate characteristics coupled with cystoscopy provide data to guide the decision for downsizing [6, 7]. Improvement in urinary symptoms may be documented after downsizing by repeat urodynamic measures.

The PSA of 10 ng/mL is consistent with a large gland size but also possible significant tumor volume [8]. Determining the number and distribution of positive cores will provide an estimate of location and size of tumor. Additionally, multiparametric magnetic resonance (mpMRI) can be utilized to correlate with the pathology data and identify areas of tumor with reasonable accuracy [9]. Local control of tumor by ablative techniques is dependent tumor location and gland size as well as traditional factors of tumor grade and stage. It is important to note that some radiation and ablative therapies may not treat large glands completely, leading to incomplete therapies in some cases with a risk for residual tumor [10–12].

Therapeutic Management

A 60 cm^3 prostate with significant associated lower urinary tract symptoms (LUTS) will be best treated with downsizing prior to therapy. This may be accomplished with hormonal downsizing, surgical downsizing, or both. Should the patient choose radiation therapy, hormonal downsizing may be preferable to avoid the increased risk of postsurgical urinary incontinence. External beam radiation (XRT) has been employed successfully in patients with variable gland sizes, but when a large gland (60 cm^3 or greater) is associated with significant symptoms (AUA score > 20), urinary retention and irritative symptoms can be very troublesome [13]. Radiation therapy without gland downsizing is not favored in this instance. Prostate downsizing prior to radiation therapy is usually hormonally based, utilizing luteinizing hormone-releasing hormone (LHRH) analogs or 5-alpha reductase inhibitors such as finasteride or dutasteride. An approximate 25–30% reduction in prostate volume can be realized with this approach [14].

Hormonal therapy is also favored over endosurgical procedures for cryotherapy candidates [10]. This avoids the difficulties of cryo-needle placement postendosurgical resection in addition to avoiding an increased risk of urinary incontinence in patients who have undergone bladder neck resection during transurethral resection or enucleation of the prostate.

Hormonal therapy can be combined with surgical tissue reduction prior to HIFU (Table 6.1). This offers the advantage of prostate downsizing and improved urinary function prior to HIFU and renders the prostate suitable for treatment within the

Table 6.1 The contribution of transurethral resection to the reduction of morbidity of HIFU prostate ablation is demonstrated

	HIFU monotherapy ($n = 450$) 1996–1999	TURP + HIFU in 1 session ($n = 595$) since 2000	TURP 1 month before HIFU ($n = 315$) since 2003
Obstruction time (days after HIFU)	35 (epicystostomia)	9 (epicyst. + urethral)	5 (urethral)
Obstruction by necrosis and/or stenosis	34% (necrotic tissue)	9.7% (necr. + bladder neck)	8.5% (bladder neck)
Any incontinence symptoms	28% (urge + stress)	7.8% (stress only)	4.2% (stress only)
Secondary urinary tract infections	42% (no antibiotics)	12.6% (1 week antibiotics)	6.4% (1 week antibiotics)
Rectourethral fistula	4% ($n = 18$)	0% ($n = 0$)	0.3% ($n = 1$)
Tissue sludging	75%	12.6%	4/2%
Any of these side effects per patient	100%	42.7%	25.4%

From Thuroff, S. and C. Chaussy, *Evolution and outcomes of 3 MHz high intensity focused ultrasound therapy for localized prostate cancer during 15 years.* J Urol, 2013. **190**(2): p. 702–10, with permission

limits of the HIFU device ultrasonic beam [15, 16]. Repeat prostate ultrasound may be needed to confirm sufficient reduction in prostate height if hormonal therapy alone is selected.

When hormonal downsizing alone is not likely to reduce prostate gland size sufficiently, endosurgical techniques such as transurethral resection or laser enucleation may be employed for relief of bladder outlet obstruction prior to and after radiation or ablative therapies [16].

Should a pretreatment prostate resection be contemplated with any of the ablative techniques, it is important to recognize the critical role of the intrinsic urethral sphincter in maintaining urinary continence after bladder neck resection. It is therefore extremely important to avoid overtreatment of the prostate apex during XRT, brachytherapy, cryotherapy, or HIFU procedures in patients patients' status post endosurgical resection as the bladder neck is likely defunctionalized.

Resection of bladder neck tissues and prostate lobes prior to radiation therapy does increase the risk for urinary incontinence and should be performed judiciously to only improve voiding and not for aggressive size reduction. Bladder neck resection may be a necessary component of any endosurgical resection for symptom relief, however. Endosurgical resection performed after prostate radiation can be associated with a 50% risk of urinary incontinence, presumably due to intrinsic urethral sphincter incompetence from radiation-induced fibrosis [17]. Transurethral resection of the prostate (TURP) or laser enucleation is optimal if completed in advance of radiation treatments and does not include extensive bladder neck resection.

Brachytherapy is ideally employed in prostates 40 cm^3 or less, mostly to avoid problems with urinary retention and urethral stricture posttreatment [18].

Downsizing may be helpful in patients undergoing radioactive seed implantation (brachytherapy). TURP or enucleation prior to brachytherapy may complicate the placement of radioactive material and the retention of this radioactive material (seeds). For this reason, endosurgical resection of the prostate prior to brachytherapy is not a preferred choice for downsizing in some patients [19].

In cryotherapy-treated patients, resection of the prostate gland may complicate cryo-needle placement. In addition, despite the use of a urethral warming urinary catheter, however, sloughing of tissue may still occur with cryotherapy. This may result in an increase in obstructive urinary symptoms. For this reason, large glands >60 cm^3 are not optimal for cryotherapy but can be pretreated with hormonal downsizing techniques to bring the gland to an optimal size. This is commonly employed as a preparative measure prior to treatment [10].

In HIFU-treated patients, no cooling of the urethra occurs during treatment, and urethral tissues are included in the thermal zone of tissue coagulation. These patients may experience significant sloughing of tissue post-HIFU. Post-HIFU urinary retention may persist after catheter removal. Treatment via endoscopic resection of prostatic lobe and bladder neck tissue prior to HIFU therapy alleviates this problem in a majority of cases [16]. Endoscopic tissue reduction may also remove significant amounts of gland rendering the prostate within range of the focused ultrasound energy beam. Downsizing of the prostate prior to HIFU serves a dual purpose of alleviating symptoms, as well preparing the prostate for whole gland therapy. The limit of the HIFU ultrasonic beam energy delivered by the current FDA-approved HIFU devices in the United States is approximately 25–30 mm in the anterior-posterior dimension [2].

Prostate downsizing can affect serum PSA levels. Monitoring of therapeutic success post radiation or ablation must take into account the effect of prostate tissue reduction surgery or hormonal downsizing on PSA. While prostate-specific antigen (PSA) values decline significantly with hormonal therapy, TURP may also significantly reduce PSA levels as well. On average, TURP for voiding improvement results in up to a 50–90% decline in PSA compared to pre-surgical levels [20]. Determining a new baseline PSA pre- and post-therapy is a key step in establishing accurate PSA monitoring and cancer surveillance. Pretreatment PSA and PSA monitoring every 6 months after radiation or ablative therapy provides a point of comparison for determining response and cancer control [11].

In addition to PSA testing, imaging can be useful for monitoring response to treatment. The use of prostate mpMRI as a monitoring tool remains formative at this time and will require further refinement before becoming widely accepted. Nonetheless, prostate multi-parametric magnetic resonance imaging (mpMRI) in selected patients may accurately define treated areas of the prostate and be useful for serial imaging and detection of recurrence. This technology is not employed post-radiation routinely, but it is promising for cryotherapy and HIFU patients [21, 22]. Prostate mpMRI pre-cryotherapy or pre-HIFU may be repeated at 6–12 months post-therapy to confirm adequate treatment effect in the target zone and for future imaging comparisons.

Conclusion

A 74-year-old male patient with a 60 cm^3 enlarged prostate and significant voiding symptoms desires a therapy that is not a radical surgery. Whether this patient chooses radiation therapy or an ablative therapy, his large, symptomatic prostate will be a complicating factor for treatment of his prostate cancer. With adequate gland preparation, however, he may be successfully treated with greater comfort and efficacy if downsizing techniques are employed. These therapies may be hormonal, endosurgical, or both in combination. Urodynamic assessment, PSA monitoring, and MRI imaging may be useful adjuncts to a basic downsizing strategy. Cancer control and functional preservation and improvement represent the combined goals of this approach.

References

1. Roberts CB, et al. Treatment profile and complications associated with cryotherapy for localized prostate cancer: a population-based study. Prostate Cancer Prostatic Dis. 2011;14(4):313–9.
2. Thuroff S, Chaussy C. Evolution and outcomes of 3 MHz high intensity focused ultrasound therapy for localized prostate cancer during 15 years. J Urol. 2013;190(2):702–10.
3. Tacklind J, et al. Finasteride for benign prostatic hyperplasia. Cochrane Database Syst Rev. 2010;(10):CD006015.
4. Baten E, van Renterghem K. The advantages of transurethral resection of the prostate in patients with an elevated or rising prostate specific antigen, mild or moderate lower urinary tract symptoms, bladder outlet obstruction and negative prostate cancer imaging or prostate biopsies: a prospective analysis in 105 consecutive patients. Curr Urol. 2017;10(3):140–4.
5. Kuebker JM, Miller NL. Holmium laser enucleation of the prostate: patient selection and outcomes. Curr Urol Rep. 2017;18(12):96.
6. Rutman MP, Blaivas JG. Urodynamics: what to do and when is it clinically necessary? Curr Urol Rep. 2007;8(4):263–8.
7. Blaivas JG, Weiss JP. Benign prostatic hyperplasia and lower urinary tract symptoms. Preface. Urol Clin North Am. 2009;36(4):xi–xiii.
8. Nordstrom T, et al. Prostate-specific antigen (PSA) density in the diagnostic algorithm of prostate cancer. Prostate Cancer Prostatic Dis. 2017.
9. Bjurlin MA, et al. Prediction of prostate cancer risk among men undergoing combined MRI-targeted and systematic biopsy using novel pre-biopsy nomograms that incorporate MRI findings. Urology. 2017.
10. Tay KJ, et al. Primary cryotherapy for high-grade clinically localized prostate cancer: oncologic and functional outcomes from the COLD registry. J Endourol. 2016;30(1):43–8.
11. Crouzet S, et al. Whole-gland ablation of localized prostate cancer with high-intensity focused ultrasound: oncologic outcomes and morbidity in 1002 patients. Eur Urol. 2014;65(5):907–14.
12. Braunstein LZ, et al. Whole pelvis versus prostate-only radiotherapy with or without short-course androgen deprivation therapy and mortality risk. Clin Genitourin Cancer. 2015;13(6):555–61.
13. Kim S, et al. Severe genitourinary toxicity following radiation therapy for prostate cancer—how long does it last? J Urol. 2013;189(1):116–21.
14. Kumar S, et al. Neo-adjuvant and adjuvant hormone therapy for localised and locally advanced prostate cancer. Cochrane Database Syst Rev. 2006;(4):CD006019.

15. Hatiboglu G, et al. Quality of life and functional outcome after infravesical desobstruction and HIFU treatment for localized prostate cancer. BMC Urol. 2017;17(1):5.
16. Netsch C, Pfeiffer D, Gross AJ. Development of bladder outlet obstruction after a single treatment of prostate cancer with high-intensity focused ultrasound: experience with 226 patients. J Endourol. 2010;24(9):1399–403.
17. Ishiyama H, et al. Is there an increase in genitourinary toxicity in patients treated with transurethral resection of the prostate and radiotherapy? A systematic review. Am J Clin Oncol. 2014;37(3):297–304.
18. Thomas MD, et al. Identifying the predictors of acute urinary retention following magnetic-resonance-guided prostate brachytherapy. Int J Radiat Oncol Biol Phys. 2000;47(4):905–8.
19. Stone NN, Ratnow ER, Stock RG. Prior transurethral resection does not increase morbidity following real-time ultrasound-guided prostate seed implantation. Tech Urol. 2000;6(2):123–7.
20. Dutkiewicz S, Stepien K. Serum PSA levels at 6 month after surgery, TURP or Doxazosin therapy for BPH. Mater Med Pol. 1996;28(2):69–70.
21. Martino P, et al. Role of imaging and biopsy to assess local recurrence after definitive treatment for prostate carcinoma (surgery, radiotherapy, cryotherapy, HIFU). World J Urol. 2011;29(5):595–605.
22. Rouviere O. Imaging techniques for local recurrence of prostate cancer: for whom, why and how? Diagn Interv Imaging. 2012;93(4):279–90.

Chapter 7
Adjuvant Radiation Therapy for High-Risk Post-prostatectomy Patients

William C. Jackson, Daniel E. Spratt, and Todd M. Morgan

Clinical Case Scenario: 70-year-old man status post radical prostatectomy for Gleason score 8 (4 + 4) prostate cancer. Pathology revealed pT3aN0M0 disease with a focal positive bladder neck margin. His PSA is undetectable 8 weeks postoperatively. He would like to consider adjuvant radiation therapy.

Radical prostatectomy is increasingly utilized as the initial definitive treatment for men with high-risk prostate cancer and is currently the most common initial treatment modality for this group of men in the United States [1, 2]. As the number of men undergoing radical prostatectomy for high-risk disease increases, so too does the number of men with potentially adverse postoperative pathologic findings such as a positive surgical margin (+SM), extraprostatic extension (EPE), or seminal vesicle invasion (SVI) [3]. Based on results from three randomized clinical trials assessing adjuvant radiation therapy (ART) following radical prostatectomy [4–7], national guidelines from the American Urological Association (AUA) and American Society for Radiation Oncology (ASTRO) state that "physicians should offer adjuvant radiotherapy to patients with adverse pathologic findings at prostatectomy," where adverse pathologic findings are defined by the presence of a + SM, EPE, and/ or SVI. The American Society of Clinical Oncology (ASCO) has endorsed these guidelines, emphasizing the need for shared decision-making between physician and patient [8]. Despite these recommendations, less than 10% of men with any of

W. C. Jackson, M.D. · D. E. Spratt, M.D.
Department of Radiation Oncology, University of Michigan, Ann Arbor, MI, USA
e-mail: wcj@med.umich.edu; sprattda@med.umich.edu

T. M. Morgan, M.D. (✉)
Department of Urology, University of Michigan, Ann Arbor, MI, USA
e-mail: tomorgan@med.umich.edu

© Springer International Publishing AG, part of Springer Nature 2018   81
S. S. Chang, M. S. Cookson (eds.), *Prostate Cancer*,
https://doi.org/10.1007/978-3-319-78646-9_7

these three adverse pathologic features following radical prostatectomy receive ART [9–11]. This discordance is likely multifactorial in nature, including differing interpretation of the published literature surrounding ART by physicians, concerns for additive treatment-related toxicity, overtreatment of patients potentially cured by surgery, and individual patient preferences. A web-based survey assessing beliefs and practices of ART among urologists and radiation oncologists highlights that radiation oncologists are significantly more likely than urologists to recommend ART based on the presence of +SM, EPE, or SVI alone (78% vs. 44%) [12]. Notably, overall, 68% of physicians in this survey responded recommending ART based on the presence of any adverse pathologic feature; however, with a less than 10% utilization rate, these beliefs are markedly discordant with clinical practice.

For the presented clinical case with EPE and a focally positive margin, we are in agreement with national guidelines and recommend shared decision-making around the role of ART as an integral component of this patient's management. This discussion should highlight the patient's risk of biochemical recurrence in the absence of ART, the potential benefits and risks associated with ART, as well as the alternative of close PSA monitoring and early salvage radiotherapy (SRT) if indicated. In this chapter, we will discuss how to estimate a man's preoperative risk of adverse pathologic features at prostatectomy in order to facilitate early discussions of the possible role of ART. We will then review how to evaluate a patient's risk for recurrent disease following prostatectomy, transitioning to a discussion on the data supporting the role of post-prostatectomy radiation therapy for patients at high risk of local recurrence. This will lead to a summary of the debate regarding the relative efficacy of early salvage radiation therapy (eSRT) and ongoing clinical trials comparing ART to eSRT. We finally evaluate the possible role of treatment intensification for select high-risk men and close with our conclusions and recommendations for the presented clinical case.

Pre-prostatectomy Patient Evaluation

Given the endorsement for the consideration of ART for men with EPE, SVI, or +SM following radical prostatectomy by national guidelines, the pre-prostatectomy patient evaluation is critical. Men need to be appropriately counselled at the time of their initial diagnosis regarding their risk of adverse pathologic features at prostatectomy as well as the potential impact that these features may have on the possible need for subsequent therapy if they chose surgery as their primary management.

For a man considering prostatectomy, the pre-prostatectomy evaluation includes a digital rectal exam of the prostate for clinical staging, assessment of the serum prostate-specific antigen (PSA) level, and assessment of their prostate needle biopsy to determine the International Society of Urological Pathology (ISUP) grade group and approximate disease volume [13]. For men with clinical T3 or T4 disease, Gleason score $\geq$ 8 (ISUP grade group $\geq$4), PSA > 10–20 ng/mL, or nomogram-based probability of lymph node involvement >10–15%, a staging bone scan and/or pelvic CT or MRI may also be indicted to rule out the presence of metastatic disease. While clinical staging is a critical component of the initial patient evaluation, the DRE lacks both sensitivity and specificity, and a large proportion of men may be upstaged or downstaged following prostatectomy. Multiple nomograms have been created in an attempt to better estimate a man's risk of EPE, SVI, and/or lymph node involvement (LNI) at the time of prostatectomy. The Partin tables estimate a man's likelihood of having organ-confined disease and risk of EPE, SVI, and LNI based on PSA, highest biopsy Gleason score, and clinical stage [3, 14]. Using PSA and biopsy Gleason score alone, the Roach equations estimate the risk of SVI, LNI, and EPE [15–17]. Additionally, the Kattan preoperative nomogram [18], a version of which can be used online through Memorial Sloan Kettering Cancer Center's website, utilizes PSA, clinical stage, and Gleason score to estimate the likelihood of organ-confined disease, EPE, SVI, and LNI, as well as the 5- and 10-year progression-free probability after radical prostatectomy. Ten- and 15-year probabilities of cancer-specific survival after radical prostatectomy are also estimated. Tools such as these are invaluable resources to the clinician and should be utilized in shared decision-making with patients.

Returning to the 70-year-old man from the presented clinical case, if we assume that he presented with cT1c disease and a PSA of 4.0 ng/mL with 3 of 12 biopsy cores positive and a highest Gleason score of 4 + 4 = 8, the Kattan/MSKCC nomogram predicts a 63% likelihood of EPE and an 11% likelihood of SVI at prostatectomy. Conversely, if the patient presented with cT2c disease, a PSA of 10.0 ng/mL, and 9 of 12 biopsy cores positive with a highest Gleason score of 4 + 4 = 8, his predicted risk of EPE and SVI increased to 88% and 52%, respectively. In both scenarios, if the patient is most interested in pursuing definitive local therapy with radical prostatectomy, his predicted risk of EPE is >50%, and as such, he should preoperatively be counselled on the potential role of ART. Furthermore, in the second clinical scenario where the patient presents with higher baseline risk features, the MSKCC nomogram predicts a 5-year progression-free probability of only 23% following radical prostatectomy as compared to 61% in the more favorable clinical scenario. In the second scenario, the low likelihood of cure with single modality treatment should be discussed with the patient to further guide treatment decision-making. For patients with a high risk of progression following RP, it is critical to discuss the need for multimodality therapy prior to making initial management decisions.

In addition to the clinical exam and prognostic nomograms, multiparametric MRI and tissue biomarkers have emerged as potentially useful methods for disease assessment prior to definitive treatment. A meta-analysis assessing the diagnostic accuracy of MR imaging for local staging of prostate cancer in 75 studies with 9796 patients showed a specificity of 91%, 96%, and 88% for detecting EPE, SVI, and overall presence of stage T3 disease, respectively [19]. The sensitivity of MR imaging to rule out the presence of any of these features was dramatically lower, ranging from 57 to 61% [19]. Thus, while there is a strong correlation between the presence of EPE and SVI on multiparametric MRI and final post-prostatectomy pathology, the absence of these features on multiparametric MRI by no means excludes the possibility of their presence on final pathology.

Finally, tissue-based molecular classifiers can aid in estimating the risk of adverse pathology and/or long-term progression following RP [20–22]. OncotypeDx Prostate, Decipher, and Prolaris each assess the expression of a different set of genes and are commercially available for interrogation of biopsy tissue [20–24].

In summary, for men undergoing prostatectomy, a standard clinical evaluation can be coupled with prognostic nomograms, multiparametric MRI, and/or tissue-based molecular classifiers to help estimate a man's likelihood of having EPE or SVI at prostatectomy. The risk of adverse pathologic features can thereby guide preoperative discussions, including the possible role of postoperative RT.

Post-prostatectomy Patient Evaluation

For men undergoing prostatectomy for treatment of localized prostate cancer, such as the patient in the presented case scenario, postoperative evaluation should initially focus on the patient's recovery from surgery. Attention should then shift to estimating the man's risk of future disease progression in the absence of additional therapy, and weighing this risk against the patient's predicted life expectancy, as adjuvant local therapy is typically not recommended for men with a life expectancy <10 years. Most commonly, recurrent prostate cancer following prostatectomy is initially detected by a rise in PSA. Following prostatectomy, men should experience a PSA nadir to <0.1 ng/mL, which is considered undetectable. While the lower limits of any given PSA assay can vary, and ultrasensitive PSA tests can detect PSA in quantities as low as 0.01 ng/mL, the <0.1 ng/mL threshold is generally considered the standard. As the half-life of serum PSA is 2 to 3 days, the initial post-prostatectomy PSA should not be assessed until at least 3 weeks postoperatively (7 half-lives to allow for 99% elimination). Men with a persistently detectable PSA ≥ 0.1 ng/mL constitute a distinct cohort and will be discussed later.

There are numerous definitions of biochemically recurrent prostate cancer (BCR), but a common definition and the one utilized by the AUA is a PSA value of 0.2 ng/mL followed by a second confirmatory level of 0.2 ng/mL or higher [25]. For men with an undetectable post-prostatectomy PSA, long-term rates of BCR following radical prostatectomy vary depending on the risk profile of the cohort, but generally range from 20 to 40% [26–28]. Modern series suggest that the risk of BCR exceeds 50% for men with high-risk prostate cancer undergoing prostatectomy [29, 30]. Based on these numbers, it is estimated that approximately 14,000–27,000 men per year will develop biochemically recurrent prostate cancer (Fig. 7.1) [1, 11, 31–35]. At least one-third of these will go on to develop metastatic disease [27, 36]. Given the large number of men at risk for disease progression following radical prostatectomy, there has been significant interest in identifying the highest risk men for consideration of adjuvant therapy in an attempt to reduce the rate of recurrence.

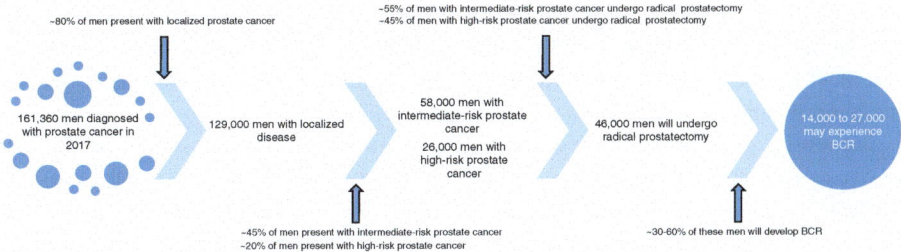

Fig. 7.1 Approximation of the number of men at risk annually for biochemical recurrence following radical prostatectomy in the United States. *BCR* biochemical recurrence

Several pathologic features following prostatectomy are associated with an increased risk for development of BCR including histology, Gleason score, the presence of a positive surgical margin, EPE, SVI, and LNI [37–42]. The vast majority of prostate cancers are adenocarcinomas or variants of adenocarcinoma [43, 44]. Approximately 5% are non-adenocarcinoma variants. Certain histologic subtypes are known to portend a poor prognosis, such as the ductal and intraductal adenocarcinomas, as well as the neuroendocrine histology small cell carcinoma [43, 45]. Additionally, prostate cancers arising in the setting of a germline BRCA2 mutation appear to be more aggressive [46]. Despite the poorer prognosis associated with these rare histologies, data are lacking to support altering clinical management based on their presence. The Gleason score has consistently been demonstrated to be the single most prognostic pathologic feature in prostate cancer. The presence of Gleason pattern 5 (ISUP grade group 5) disease confers a low likelihood of cure with single modality treatment, with 5-year rates of BCR following prostatectomy approaching 75% [30]. Overall, the 5-year rates of BCR following radical prostatectomy for ISUP grade groups 1, 2, 3, 4, and 5 are approximately 4%, 12%, 37%, 52%, and 74% [30], emphasizing the prognostic importance of the Gleason score. The presence of a + SM, EPE, SVI, or involved pelvic lymph nodes have all been shown to independently predict an increased risk of recurrence following prostatectomy as well [41].

Just as there are nomograms to predict a man's progression-free survival prior to prostatectomy, as previously discussed, there are postoperative tools available that incorporate the valuable prognostic information gained following surgery to help estimate man's future risk of disease recurrence. The most commonly utilized aids include the Stephenson nomogram, a version of which is available through the Memorial Sloan Kettering Cancer Center website, and the CAPRA-S score [41, 47, 48]. The postoperative Stephenson nomogram utilizes surgical margin status; presence of EPE, SVI, and LNI; Gleason score; pre-operative PSA; and number of months free of disease after radical prostatectomy to estimate a patient's 10-year progression-free probability. Similarly, the CAPRA-S score is a simple calculation determined using patients' pre-prostatectomy PSA; surgical margin status; presence of SVI, EPE, or LNI; and Gleason score to derive a score from 0 to 12. Each scoring increment is associated with an increased 5-year risk of biochemical progression.

Overall, the most adverse pathologic features in these models are a Gleason score of 8 or higher and the presence of SVI, EPE, or a + SM. The presence of LNI is likely the most ominous prognostic pathologic finding despite a lower relative weight in each model and is considered a stage IV disease.

Recently, prostatectomy specimen-based genomic classifiers that can further assist in risk stratifying men following radical prostatectomy have entered into clinical practice. The most utilized to date is the Decipher score, an RNA expression-based molecular classifier shown to be independently associated with the risk of metastasis and prostate cancer-specific mortality [23, 24]. This test provides a score of 0 to 1, with a score of 0–0.45 categorized as low-risk, 0.45–0.6 average risk, and 0.6–1.0 high-risk of developing metastatic disease within 5 years and of dying from prostate cancer within 10 years in the absence of any additional treatment following prostatectomy. An individual patient-level meta-analysis of this 22-marker test found that the 10-year cumulative rates of metastatic disease for men with low-, intermediate-, and high-risk classification were 5.5%, 15%, and 26.7%, respectively [24]. Surveys of board-certified urologists and radiation oncologists indicate that the additional prognostic information provided might alter physician treatment recommendations in up to 30–40% of patient cases [49–51].

To summarize, clinical, pathologic, and genomic information can be utilized when estimating a man's risk for disease recurrence following prostatectomy. The pathologic features that are most prognostic for future recurrence include a Gleason score of 8 or higher (ISUP grade group ≥4) and the presence of SVI, EPE, or a + SM. Genomic classifiers can further improve discrimination in identifying men at highest risk of recurrence. Once again considering the clinical case presented in this chapter, this 70-year-old man has multiple high-risk pathologic findings that place him at a substantial risk for future BCR including EPE, a + SM, and a Gleason score of 4 + 4 = 8. He has an undetectable PSA 8 weeks postoperatively. If we assume a preoperative PSA of 7 ng/mL, the Memorial Sloan Kettering/Stephenson nomogram predicts 5- and 10-year recurrence rates of 73% and 85%, respectively. His 15-year risk of dying from prostate cancer is estimated at 8%. Given the high predicted probability of disease recurrence within 5 years, the use of adjuvant radiotherapy is appropriate to reduce his risk of recurrence and provides guideline-concordant care.

Post-prostatectomy Radiation Therapy

Post-prostatectomy radiation therapy is most commonly delivered in one of two clinical scenarios, both with curative intent: (1) as planned adjuvant therapy in the setting of adverse pathologic features and an undetectable PSA or (2) as salvage therapy in the setting of a detectable/rising PSA, with or without a clinically detectable (i.e., radiographic or palpable) prostate bed recurrence.

Adjuvant Radiation Therapy

Based on the substantial risk for disease recurrence in men undergoing prostatectomy found to have adverse pathologic features, three independent phase 3 randomized clinical trials have assessed ART in this setting: Southwest Oncology Group (SWOG) 8794, European Organisation for Research and Treatment of Cancer (EORTC) 22911, and Arbeitsgemeinschaft Radiologische Onkologie (ARO) 9602 [4–6], all of which have greater than 10 years of posttreatment follow-up. Table 7.1 summarizes the inclusion criteria and notable outcomes for these trials. All three trials have limited enrollment to men with pathologic T3 disease (EPE or SVI) and/ or positive surgical margins. In total, these trials demonstrate for men with any of these three adverse pathologic features, that on average, immediate postoperative ART reduces the risk of future BCR by approximately half compared to observation. This improvement in BCR was realized through improved locoregional control associated with ART [5, 52].

While all three trials demonstrated similar improvement in biochemical control, there are several key differences between the trials. Approximately one third of men on SWOG 8794 and EORTC 22911 had detectable post-prostatectomy PSA values, whereas these men were excluded from ARO 9602. Men with a detectable post-prostatectomy PSA have inferior long-term outcomes compared to men with an undetectable PSA, and receipt of radiation therapy in the setting of a persistently positive PSA is currently considered salvage radiation therapy (SRT), thus making ARO 9602 the only trial to have an experimental arm composed completely of true ART. Additionally, approximately 33% of men on the control arms in both SWOG 8794 and EORTC 22911 received SRT after BCR. Consequently, in modern terminology, these two trials were in essence a comparison of ART and SRT to late SRT or observation. Additionally, the SWOG and EORTC trials were both initiated before routine use of screening PSA. As such, the men on these trials likely had more advanced disease at the time of prostatectomy than many men today would.

Perhaps the most important question, though, is whether ART decreases the rate of metastasis and death for patients at high risk of local recurrence, and the SWOG and EORTC differ with respect to these endpoints. SWOG 8794 found that treatment with ART resulted in a statistically significant 10% improvement in metastasis-free survival 10 years posttreatment, which translated to an improvement in overall survival. Conversely, EORTC 22911 demonstrated no improvement in MFS or OS associated with receipt of ART. ARO 9602 was not powered to assess any endpoint other than BCR. There are several potential explanations for the discrepant MFS findings in the SWOG and EORTC trials. First, 10-year overall survival in the control arm was markedly lower on SWOG 8794 than EORTC 22911 (66% vs. 81%), indicating that men in the SWOG trial may have had more aggressive disease than those in the EORTC trial. Indeed, more men on SWOG 8794 had SVI (33% vs. 26%), and more men had all three adverse pathologic features present (22% vs. 12%). Second, differences in utilization and timing of salvage therapies in the control arms may have also contributed. Overall, patients were seen in follow-up more

Table 7.1 Prospective randomized clinical trials assessing adjuvant radiation therapy (ART)

Trial	Enrollment period	Median follow-up	Inclusion criteria	Treatment arms	Primary outcome	Patients	% detectable PSA at ART	SVI	EPE	SM+	EPE+/ SVI+/ SM+	bPFS	MFS	OS	Salvage RT	Salvage ADT
SWOG 8794	1988–1997	12.6 years	pT3 or +SM	60–64 Gy vs. Observation	MFS	425	33% >0.2 ng/mL	33%	67% with EPE or +SM and no SVI		22.1%	10 years ~53% vs. ~25%	10 years 71% vs. 61%	10 years 74% vs. 66%	33%	By 5 years 10% vs. 21%
EORTC 22911	1992–2001	10.6 years	pT3 or +SM	60 Gy vs. Observation	bPFS	1005	30.5% >0.2 ng/mL	25.5%	77.0%	62.6%	12.3%	10 years 60.6% vs. 41.1%	10 years 76.5% vs. 71.3%	10 years 76.9% vs. 80.7%	33%	By 5 years 10.1% vs. 15.5%
ARO 9602	1997–2004	9.3 years	pT3–4 or +SM	60 Gy vs. Observation	bPFS	307	0%	27%	65%	64%	NR	10 years 56% vs. 35%	NR	10 years 86% vs. 83%	NR	By 5 years 8% vs.16%

ART, adjuvant radiation therapy; PSA, prostate-specific antigen; SVI, seminal vesicle invasion; EPE, extraprostatic extension; SM+, positive surgical margin; bPFS, biochemical progression-free survival; MFS, metastasis-free survival; OS, overall survival; ADT, androgen deprivation therapy frequently on the EORTC study, and a more stringent definition of BCR was employed (two consecutive PSA values >0.2 ng/mL vs. increase in postoperative PSA to >0.4 ng/mL). Furthermore, while the percentage of patients receiving SRT in the control arm was 33% in both trials, a larger proportion of men experienced BCR in the SWOG trial, meaning that the overall utilization of SRT in this trial was lower than in the EORTC trial. In summary, there is strong level one evidence that ART following prostatectomy for men with adverse pathologic features reduces the risk of BCR by half, but the impact of ART on metastasis and OS relative to SRT is still an open question.

When considering the clinical benefits of ART, one must carefully weigh the potential associated toxicities and impact on patient quality of life. Acute treatment-related urinary and bowel toxicity is common during and following ART, although usually mild in nature. Severe acute toxicity secondary to ART is rare. On EORTC 22911 3.1% of patients required a radiation treatment break secondary to acute toxicities, which were most commonly loose stools or increased urinary frequency. Very few men had acute grade 3+ symptoms (5.3% grade 3 loose stools, 4.4% grade 3 urinary frequency or dysuria). ART results in an increase in overall cumulative incidence of toxicities of any grade with a 23.8% vs. 11.9% rate for ART versus observation on SWOG 8794 ($p = 0.002$) and 21.9% in the RT arm versus 3.7% in the wait-and-see group on ARO 9602. Late ART-related toxicity was low on all three trials. On EORTC 22911 there was a slight increase in late grade 3+ toxicity associated with ART (5.3% vs. 2.5%). Urethral stricture was more common for men receiving ART, occurring in 17.8% of men receiving ART compared to 9.5% of observed men on SWOG 8794. Late toxicity was even less common on ARO 9602 with only 6 patients in total experiencing a late grade 2+ toxicity and only 1 man developing a urinary stricture. The very low rates of late toxicity on this trial may be secondary to improved surgical and radiation techniques, as ARO 9602 was initiated almost a decade after SWOG 8794. SWOG 8794 uniquely recorded and analyzed patient-reported health-related quality of life (HRQOL) [53]. These data demonstrated that ART resulted in an acute decline in bowel HRQOL which nearly resolved within 2 years, as well as persistently worse urinary frequency HRQOL overtime. ART was not associated with worsening erectile dysfunction HRQOL. Despite the transient decline in bowel HRQOL and persistent and stable decline in urinary frequency HRQOL, ART was associated with better global HRQOL 2-year posttreatment than surgery alone, possibly secondary to prevention of disease recurrence and avoidance of salvage therapies.

Salvage Radiation Therapy

Fundamentally, concerns for overtreatment exist if ART were to be given to all men with adverse pathologic factors following radical prostatectomy. A substantial proportion of men with one or multiple adverse pathologic features will never develop a rise in PSA following prostatectomy, as evident in the control arms from the three randomized ART trials. If treated, these men are unnecessarily at risk of short- and long-term treatment-related toxicities from ART with no potential for improved disease control. The concern for overtreatment and the fact that only one of the three randomized trials demonstrated an improvement in any endpoint other than BCR has resulted in the low utilization of ART in the United States, with many physicians preferring a more selective approach centered around salvage radiotherapy for patients with BCR. Even though this approach is favored, practice pattern data suggest that SRT is also underutilized [9].

Unfortunately, there are currently no randomized data comparing ART with selective SRT for patients with early BCR. Instead, support for SRT is derived from well-performed retrospective analyses. Trock et al. reported on 635 men who had previously undergone radical prostatectomy and then developed BCR, with 397 men receiving no salvage treatment and 238 receiving SRT [54]. With 6 years of follow-up, SRT was independently associated with a threefold improvement in prostate cancer-specific survival for men with a PSA doubling time < 6 months. A similar analysis performed by Cotter et al., but with 11 years of follow-up, assessed 519 men with post-prostatectomy BCR. SRT was administered to 158 and was associated with improved all-cause survival independent of PSADT, indicating that men with both indolent and aggressive recurrences may benefit from SRT [55]. These analyses suggest that a proportion of men with recurrent disease following prostatectomy can be cured with the use of SRT.

SRT is given with the assumption that BCR occurs secondary to locally recurrent disease in the prostate bed; however, a minority of men receiving SRT will be cured, possibly secondary to the presence of micrometastatic disease distant to the radiation treatment field at the time of SRT. Stephenson et al. created the most commonly utilized nomogram to predict a man's likelihood of biochemical control following SRT, with a recent update published by Tendulkar et al. [56, 57]. These data demonstrate that risk factors for a "second biochemical failure" following SRT include an increasing pre-SRT PSA, high Gleason score, and SVI or EPE. Features that improve the likelihood of success with SRT include a positive surgical margin, as this increases the likelihood of locally recurrent disease, and the use of neoadjuvant/concurrent androgen deprivation therapy with SRT. It should be emphasized that while men with adverse pathologic features have a lower likelihood of cure with SRT, these are the men that potentially have the most to gain with SRT. SRT should thus not be withheld based solely on the presence of adverse pathologic features. The updated analysis of over 2000 men also demonstrated that contemporary radiation doses >66 Gy are more effective than lower RT doses and also, importantly, demonstrated that SRT performed at lower PSA values was associated with a lower risk of developing DM [57]. Indeed, multiple studies have demonstrated that "early SRT" (eSRT) performed at low PSA levels improves the likelihood of long-term disease control, without an apparent pre-SRT PSA threshold, and that eSRT should be defined by PSA level as opposed to time from RP [58, 59]. In total there is good evidence that SRT is most effective when delivered with a PSA value of ≤0.5 ng/mL, and a PSA threshold of ≤0.2 ng/mL may be even more beneficial.

While retrospective data support the role of eSRT for men developing BCR following RP, the critical question is whether eSRT is as effective as ART, and there are no published randomized data to answer this question. However, multiple ongoing clinical trials are currently comparing these two treatment approaches. The Radiotherapy and Androgen Deprivation in Combination After Local Surgery (RADICALS; NCT00541047) [60] trial randomizes men with adverse pathologic features to either immediate ART or eSRT at the time of BCR. The trial is also assessing the role of and duration of ADT in this same population and completed accrual in December 2016. Radiotherapy Adjuvant Versus Early Salvage (RAVES; NCT00860652) [61] similarly is comparing ART to eSRT, and GETUG-17 (NCT00667069) [62] is comparing immediate ART plus ADT to SRT + ADT. As all three trials are ongoing or recently completed accrual, it will be several years before even preliminary results are available. Until then, ART should be discussed with all patients at high risk of local recurrence based on the existing randomized trial data. If through shared decision-making a patient and physician elect to proceed with a selective salvage radiation approach, routine clinical follow-up and close PSA monitoring should be performed to allow for early SRT, as this is critical for men receiving SRT.

Selective Treatment Intensification with Post-prostatectomy Radiation Therapy

As only 50–60% of patients achieve durable long-term biochemical control following ART, and even fewer achieve this with SRT, there is ongoing interest in intensifying treatment for men at highest risk of BCR following ART or SRT in an attempt to improve long-term disease control. The best available data for treatment intensification is for the addition of ADT for some men receiving SRT. RTOG 9601 assessed the addition of 2 years of ADT (bicalutamide, 150 mg daily) to SRT and found with 10 years of follow-up that the addition of ADT improved overall survival by 5% [63]. Notably the benefit seemed to only be present among the 46% of enrolled men with a pre-SRT PSA >0.7 ng/mL, and as such these findings may not be applicable to men receiving eSRT who have a PSA < 0.5 ng/mL. GETUG-16 assessed the benefits of 6 months of ADT in a cohort of men with lower PSA values at the time of SRT, more reflective of current clinical practice than the men included on RTOG 9601 [64]. To date, only 5-year outcomes have been reported, with an 18% improvement in freedom from BCR associated with 6 months of ADT. Longer follow-up is needed to determine whether 6 months of ADT in this favorable and contemporary cohort of men receiving SRT will translate into improved outcomes in more meaningful endpoints such as distant metastases or overall survival. The ongoing RADICALS trial, previously discussed, will hopefully shed light on whether some men benefit more from the 24 months of ADT utilized in RTOG 9601 than the 6 months in GETUG-17. Until then, retrospective data suggest that men with a pre-SRT PSA $\geq$ 1.0 ng/mL or a Gleason score of 9–10 may benefit from a duration of ADT > 12 months [65]. The ongoing NRG GU-002 (NCT03070886) is assessing whether the addition of docetaxel to RT and ADT can improve outcomes for the very high-risk subset of men with a persistently elevated post-prostatectomy PSA. Finally, RTOG 0534 (NCT00567580) is assessing whether there is a benefit to radiating the pelvic lymph nodes in conjunction with the prostate bed for men receiving SRT.

RTOG 9601 and GETUG-17 demonstrate that some men receiving SRT benefit from the addition of neoadjuvant/concomitant ADT. One can hypothesize based on these findings that certain men receiving ART may also benefit from treatment intensification as well. RTOG 0621 assessed the safety and initial efficacy of the addition of ADT and docetaxel in a high-risk cohort of post-prostatectomy men receiving ART, the majority of whom had an undetectable PSA and $\geq$pT3 disease and a Gleason score $\geq$8. This study demonstrated acceptable toxicity with a 3-year freedom from progression of 73% [66], which appeared superior to historical cohorts with similar clinicopathologic features. These findings are encouraging and suggest that future randomized trials assessing the role of ADT and docetaxel in combination with ART are warranted in select men at the highest risk of future disease recurrence.

Future Directions

The ability to identify men at highest risk for residual localized prostate cancer following prostatectomy is critical when selecting men most likely to benefit from ART or eSRT. Historically, as discussed, risk of disease recurrence following prostatectomy has been estimated using clinicopathologic features and predictive nomograms. While helpful, these prognostic tools leave significant room for improvement as they fall short in their ability to identify which men are most likely to benefit from adjuvant or salvage therapy. Novel molecular imaging strategies may aid in the ability to better define which men have local and/or distant recurrences following prostatectomy. One such imaging modality is prostate-specific membrane antigen positron emission tomography (PSMA-PET). A systematic review and meta-analysis of 1309 men with recurrent prostate cancer found that 42%, 58%, 76%, and 95% of scans were positive at the corresponding PSA levels of 0–0.2, 0.2–1, 1–2, and >2 ng/mL [67]. Thus, approximately 40–50% of men with a PSA <0.5 ng/mL might be expected to have a positive finding on PSMA-PET. If the identified recurrence was outside of the pelvis, the role of SRT may be in question. Future improvements in ligand-based PET/CT imaging will likely result in improved sensitivity and specificity at lower PSA thresholds, thereby increasing clinical utility. In addition to novel imaging techniques, new molecular classifiers may also aid in identifying men most likely to benefit from post-prostatectomy radiation therapy. In a retrospective cohort of men receiving prostatectomy with or without post-prostatectomy radiation therapy, the Post-Operative Radiation Therapy Outcomes

Score (PORTOS), a 24-gene predictive biomarker, discriminated which men were most likely to benefit from post-prostatectomy radiation therapy [68]. Men with a high PORTOS score were substantially less likely to develop metastatic disease if they received post-prostatectomy RT compared to those who did not. Similarly, Den et al. retrospectively assessed the Decipher classifier in a cohort of men with pT3 or margin-positive prostate cancer who received post-prostatectomy RT (ART or SRT) [69]. Dichotomization of the classifier into high and low scores identified men who appeared to benefit from ART over SRT. Men with higher scores receiving ART had a 6% cumulative incidence of metastases at 5 years, compared to 23% for men treated with SRT. Genomic classifiers such as these may someday redefine the way in which we make decisions regarding what men should receiving post-prostatectomy radiation therapy, and whether this treatment should be delivered in the adjuvant or early salvage setting.

The Decipher score is also being assessed in an ongoing randomized controlled trial to determine its impact on physician and patient decision-making regarding the use of ART (Genomics in Michigan Impacting Observation or Radiation [G-MINOR]; NCT02783950). Men with pT3 disease or positive surgical margins following prostatectomy are randomized to either assessment of their recurrence risk using the CAPRA-S score alone or to additional risk assessment with this genomic classifier score (Fig. 7.2). Long-term results will evaluate the impact of this classifier score on the utilization of ART as well as its impact on patient outcomes.

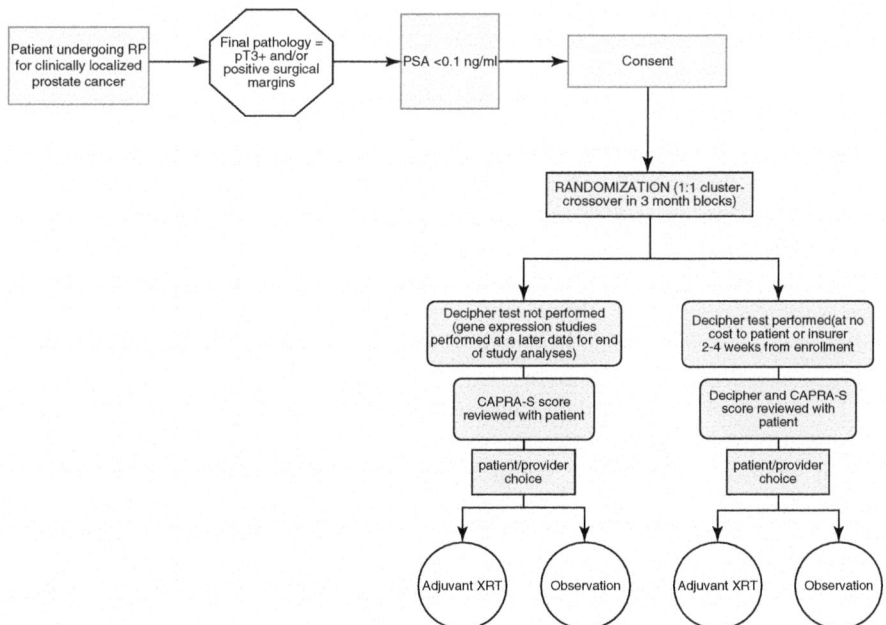

Fig. 7.2 Schema of a clinical trial (G-MINOR, NCT02783950) incorporating the Decipher score to assess its impact on physician and patient's decision-making regarding the use of adjuvant radiation therapy

Genomic classifiers are also being implemented as stratification variables on clinical trials, which will help to evaluate their ability to predict response to treatments. The Decipher score is currently a stratification variable on NRG GU-002, a phase II–III trial of adjuvant radiotherapy and androgen deprivation following radical prostatectomy with or without adjuvant docetaxel. Similarly, the PAM50 gene signature used in breast cancer was used to subtype prostate cancer into luminal A/B and basal-like subgroups, with data indicating that men with luminal-B like prostate cancer were most likely to benefit from the addition of ADT to post-prostatectomy treatment [70]. This biomarker will be used to stratify men on the upcoming NRG GU-006 randomized trial assessing the role of a second-generation antiandrogen in combination with SRT.

Endeavors evaluating novel imaging studies and genomic classifiers will continue to reshape the way in which we approach post-prostatectomy radiation therapy. The ultimate goal is to be able to identify men at the highest risk for disease recurrence who will benefit from immediate ART, those at moderate risk who can be closely observed for consideration of eSRT and thereby potentially be spared from unnecessary toxicity associated with post-prostatectomy radiation therapy, and those at low risk who can avoid the need for any additional post-prostatectomy treatment.

Conclusions and Recommendations for Presented Clinical Case

Three randomized trials demonstrate a clinical benefit associated with ART for men with pathologic T3 disease or a positive surgical margin following radical prostatectomy. Despite this benefit and national guidelines recommending offering ART to these men, utilization of ART remains low. While severe long-term toxicity secondary to ART is rare, there are warranted concerns of overtreatment, as many men with adverse pathologic features will never develop recurrent disease, and thereby have nothing to gain from additional therapy. As such, a selective salvage radiation approach is common for men with an undetectable PSA following prostatectomy. If this approach is taken, men should be followed closely to allow for consideration of eSRT, as the best available data suggest that SRT is most effective at PSA values <0.5 ng/mL, with continued improvement in outcomes at even lower PSA values. Certain men with high-risk features, including a persistently positive post-prostatectomy PSA, a PSA > 0.5 ng/mL, or Gleason score ≥ 8, may benefit from intensification of treatment with ADT or other systemic therapies at the time of ART or SRT. Utilization of genomic classifiers is increasing as they allow for improved recurrence risk estimation following prostatectomy, and they are currently used as stratification variables in clinical trials to evaluate their ability to predict response to treatment.

Returning to the clinical case presented in this chapter, this patient is a 70-year-old man status post prostatectomy with Gleason score 4 + 4 = 8 prostate cancer.

Final pathology revealed pT3aN0M0 disease with a focal positive bladder neck margin, and his PSA was subsequently undetectable 8. If we assume a preoperative PSA of 7 ng/mL, the Memorial Sloan Kettering/Stephenson nomogram predicts 5- and 10-year recurrence-free survival rates of 27% and 15%, respectively. His 15-year risk of dying from prostate cancer is estimated at 8%. Based on level one evidence, our practice is to offer ART for all men with a 10-year life expectancy who have pathologic T3 disease or a positive surgical margin, discussing the potential risks and benefits of ART in a multidisciplinary setting. For men with pathologic T3 disease or a positive surgical margin and an estimated risk of BCR > 60% at 5 years, our recommendation has generally been for ART over an eSRT-based approach. Despite being 70 years old, if his life expectancy is at least 10 years, he has a very low likelihood of remaining disease-free over this time, and based on his multiple adverse pathologic features, it is likely that there would be consideration of treatment intensification at the time of SRT, such as the addition of ADT to SRT. Assuming the patient is interested in ART, we would defer ART until his urinary recovery postoperatively had been maximized, which is often around the 6-month mark. For men with adverse pathologic features and a 5-year risk of recurrence <60%, we explain that level I evidence demonstrates that ART reduces patients' risk of a future rise in PSA by approximately 50%, but that this may or may not translate to improved survival. We also explain that there is some chance that the PSA will never rise, and therefore adjuvant therapy may be of no benefit and put the patient at risk for unnecessary treatment toxicity. In this light, we discuss the possible role of eSRT, noting the caveat that we do not yet know if this approach is as effective as ART. Men who are risk-averse to disease recurrence and less concerned about additional treatment-related toxicity may opt for ART, and we are comfortable offering this based on the existing level I evidence. We anticipate that the next several years will bring important data regarding the role of ART compared to eSRT and shed light on the optimal use of molecular classifiers in this important clinical setting.

References

1. Cooperberg MR, Carroll PR. Trends in management for patients with localized prostate cancer, 1990–2013. JAMA. 2015;314(1):80–2.
2. Weiner AB, Matulewicz RS, Schaeffer EM, Liauw SL, Feinglass JM, Eggener SE. Contemporary management of men with high-risk localized prostate cancer in the United States. Prostate Cancer Prostatic Dis. 2017;20(3):283–8.
3. Tosoian JJ, Chappidi M, Feng Z, et al. Prediction of pathological stage based on clinical stage, serum prostate-specific antigen, and biopsy Gleason score: Partin tables in the contemporary era. BJU Int. 2017;119(5):676–83.
4. Wiegel T, Bartkowiak D, Bottke D, et al. Prostate-specific antigen persistence after radical prostatectomy as a predictive factor of clinical relapse-free survival and overall survival: 10-year data of the ARO 96-02 trial. Int J Radiat Oncol Biol Phys. 2015;91(2):288–94.
5. Bolla M, van Poppel H, Tombal B, et al. Postoperative radiotherapy after radical prostatectomy for high-risk prostate cancer: long-term results of a randomised controlled trial (EORTC trial 22911). Lancet. 2012;380(9858):2018–27.

6. Thompson IM, Tangen CM, Paradelo J, et al. Adjuvant radiotherapy for pathological T3N0M0 prostate cancer significantly reduces risk of metastases and improves survival: long-term followup of a randomized clinical trial. J Urol. 2009;181(3):956–62.

7. Thompson IM, Valicenti RK, Albertsen P, et al. Adjuvant and salvage radiotherapy after prostatectomy: AUA/ASTRO guideline. J Urol. 2013;190(2):441–9.

8. Freedland SJ, Rumble RB, Finelli A, et al. Adjuvant and salvage radiotherapy after prostatectomy: American Society of Clinical Oncology clinical practice guideline endorsement. J Clin Oncol. 2014;32(34):3892–8.

9. Morgan TM, Hawken SR, Ghani KR, et al. Variation in the use of postoperative radiotherapy among high-risk patients following radical prostatectomy. Prostate Cancer Prostatic Dis. 2016;19(2):216–21.

10. Kalbasi A, Swisher-McClure S, Mitra N, et al. Low rates of adjuvant radiation in patients with nonmetastatic prostate cancer with high-risk pathologic features. Cancer. 2014;120(19):3089–96.

11. Sineshaw HM, Gray PJ, Efstathiou JA, Jemal A. Declining use of radiotherapy for adverse features after radical prostatectomy: results from the National Cancer Data Base. Eur Urol. 2015;68(5):768–74.

12. Showalter TN, Ohri N, Teti KG, et al. Physician beliefs and practices for adjuvant and salvage radiation therapy after prostatectomy. Int J Radiat Oncol Biol Phys. 2012;82(2):e233–8.

13. Epstein JI, Egevad L, Amin MB, Delahunt B, Srigley JR, Humphrey PA. The 2014 International Society of Urological Pathology (ISUP) consensus conference on Gleason grading of prostatic carcinoma: definition of grading patterns and proposal for a new grading system. Am J Surg Pathol. 2016;40(2):244–52.

14. Partin AW, Yoo J, Carter HB, et al. The use of prostate specific antigen, clinical stage and Gleason score to predict pathological stage in men with localized prostate cancer. J Urol. 1993;150(1):110–4.

15. Diaz A, Roach M 3rd, Marquez C, et al. Indications for and the significance of seminal vesicle irradiation during 3D conformal radiotherapy for localized prostate cancer. Int J Radiat Oncol Biol Phys. 1994;30(2):323–9.

16. Roach M 3rd, Marquez C, Yuo HS, et al. Predicting the risk of lymph node involvement using the pre-treatment prostate specific antigen and Gleason score in men with clinically localized prostate cancer. Int J Radiat Oncol Biol Phys. 1994;28(1):33–7.

17. Roach M 3rd, Chen A, Song J, Diaz A, Presti J Jr, Carroll P. Pretreatment prostate-specific antigen and Gleason score predict the risk of extracapsular extension and the risk of failure following radiotherapy in patients with clinically localized prostate cancer. Semin Urol Oncol. 2000;18(2):108–14.

18. Kattan MW, Eastham JA, Stapleton AMF, Wheeler TM, Scardino PT. A preoperative nomogram for disease recurrence following radical prostatectomy for prostate cancer. J Natl Cancer Inst. 1998;90(10):766–71.

19. de Rooij M, Hamoen EH, Witjes JA, Barentsz JO, Rovers MM. Accuracy of magnetic resonance imaging for local staging of prostate cancer: a diagnostic meta-analysis. Eur Urol. 2016;70(2):233–45.

20. Bishoff JT, Freedland SJ, Gerber L, et al. Prognostic utility of the cell cycle progression score generated from biopsy in men treated with prostatectomy. J Urol. 2014;192(2):409–14.

21. Cooperberg MR, Simko JP, Cowan JE, et al. Validation of a cell-cycle progression gene panel to improve risk stratification in a contemporary prostatectomy cohort. J Clin Oncol. 2013;31(11):1428–34.

22. Cullen J, Rosner IL, Brand TC, et al. A biopsy-based 17-gene genomic prostate score predicts recurrence after radical prostatectomy and adverse surgical pathology in a racially diverse population of men with clinically low- and intermediate-risk prostate cancer. Eur Urol. 2015;68(1):123–31.

23. Erho N, Crisan A, Vergara IA, et al. Discovery and validation of a prostate cancer genomic classifier that predicts early metastasis following radical prostatectomy. PLoS One. 2013;8(6):e66855.

24. Spratt DE, Yousefi K, Deheshi S, et al. Individual patient-level meta-analysis of the performance of the decipher genomic classifier in high-risk men after prostatectomy to predict development of metastatic disease. J Clin Oncol. 2017;35(18):1991.
25. Cookson MS, Aus G, Burnett AL, et al. Variation in the definition of biochemical recurrence in patients treated for localized prostate cancer: the American Urological Association Prostate Guidelines for Localized Prostate Cancer Update Panel report and recommendations for a standard in the reporting of surgical outcomes. J Urol. 2007;177(2):540–5.
26. Novara G, Ficarra V, Mocellin S, et al. Systematic review and meta-analysis of studies reporting oncologic outcome after robot-assisted radical prostatectomy. Eur Urol. 2012;62(3):382–404.
27. Pound CR, Partin AW, Eisenberger MA, Chan DW, Pearson JD, Walsh PC. Natural history of progression after PSA elevation following radical prostatectomy. JAMA. 1999;281(17):1591–7.
28. Mullins JK, Feng Z, Trock BJ, Epstein JI, Walsh PC, Loeb S. The impact of anatomical radical retropubic prostatectomy on cancer control: the 30-year anniversary. J Urol. 2012;188(6):2219–24.
29. Abdollah F, Sood A, Sammon JD, et al. Long-term cancer control outcomes in patients with clinically high-risk prostate cancer treated with robot-assisted radical prostatectomy: results from a multi-institutional study of 1100 patients. Eur Urol. 2015;68(3):497–505.
30. Epstein JI, Zelefsky MJ, Sjoberg DD, et al. A contemporary prostate cancer grading system: a validated alternative to the Gleason score. Eur Urol. 2016;69(3):428–35.
31. Banerji JS, Wolff EM, Massman JD, Odem-Davis K, Porter CR, Corman JM. Prostate needle biopsy outcomes in the era of the US preventive services task force recommendation against prostate specific antigen based screening. J Urol. 2016;195(1):66–73.
32. Gray PJ, Lin CC, Cooperberg MR, Jemal A, Efstathiou JA. Temporal trends and the impact of race, insurance, and socioeconomic status in the Management of Localized Prostate Cancer. Eur Urol. 2017;71(5):729–37.
33. Siegel RL, Miller KD, Jemal A. Cancer statistics, 2017. CA Cancer J Clin. 2017;67(1):7–30.
34. Morgan SC, Waldron TS, Eapen L, et al. Adjuvant radiotherapy following radical prostatectomy for pathologic T3 or margin-positive prostate cancer: a systematic review and meta-analysis. Radiother Oncol. 2008;88(1):1–9.
35. Dess RT, Morgan TM, Nguyen PL, et al. Adjuvant versus early salvage radiation therapy following radical prostatectomy for men with localized prostate cancer. Curr Urol Rep. 2017;18(7):55.
36. Antonarakis ES, Chen Y, Elsamanoudi SI, et al. Long-term overall survival and metastasis-free survival for men with prostate-specific antigen-recurrent prostate cancer after prostatectomy: analysis of the Center for Prostate Disease Research National Database. BJU Int. 2011;108(3):378–85.
37. Swindle P, Eastham JA, Ohori M, et al. Do margins matter? The prognostic significance of positive surgical margins in radical prostatectomy specimens. J Urol. 2008;179(5 Suppl):S47–51.
38. Epstein JI, Carmichael MJ, Pizov G, Walsh PC. Influence of capsular penetration on progression following radical prostatectomy: a study of 196 cases with long-term followup. J Urol. 1993;150(1):135–41.
39. Hull GW, Rabbani F, Abbas F, Wheeler TM, Kattan MW, Scardino PT. Cancer control with radical prostatectomy alone in 1,000 consecutive patients. J Urol. 2002;167(2 Pt 1):528–34.
40. Kattan MW, Wheeler TM, Scardino PT. Postoperative nomogram for disease recurrence after radical prostatectomy for prostate cancer. J Clin Oncol. 1999;17(5):1499.
41. Stephenson AJ, Scardino PT, Eastham JA, et al. Postoperative nomogram predicting the 10-year probability of prostate cancer recurrence after radical prostatectomy. J Clin Oncol. 2005;23(28):7005–12.
42. Epstein JI, Partin AW, Sauvageot J, Walsh PC. Prediction of progression following radical prostatectomy: a multivariate analysis of 721 men with long-term follow-up. Am J Surg Pathol. 1996;20(3):286–92.
43. Grignon DJ. Unusual subtypes of prostate cancer. Mod Pathol. 2004;17(3):316–27.
44. Humphrey PA, Moch H, Cubilla AL, Ulbright TM, Reuter VE. The 2016 WHO classification of tumours of the urinary system and male genital organs-part B: prostate and bladder tumours. Eur Urol. 2016;70(1):106–19.

45. Mazzucchelli R, Lopez-Beltran A, Cheng L, Scarpelli M, Kirkali Z, Montironi R. Rare and unusual histological variants of prostatic carcinoma: clinical significance. BJU Int. 2008;102(10):1369–74.
46. Taylor RA, Fraser M, Livingstone J, et al. Germline BRCA2 mutations drive prostate cancers with distinct evolutionary trajectories. Nat Commun. 2017;8:13671.
47. Punnen S, Freedland SJ, Presti JC Jr, et al. Multi-institutional validation of the CAPRA-S score to predict disease recurrence and mortality after radical prostatectomy. Eur Urol. 2014;65(6):1171–7.
48. Cooperberg MR, Hilton JF, Carroll PR. The CAPRA-S score: a straightforward tool for improved prediction of outcomes after radical prostatectomy. Cancer. 2011;117(22):5039–46.
49. Michalopoulos SN, Kella N, Payne R, et al. Influence of a genomic classifier on post-operative treatment decisions in high-risk prostate cancer patients: results from the PRO-ACT study. Curr Med Res Opin. 2014;30(8):1547–56.
50. Badani K, Thompson DJ, Buerki C, et al. Impact of a genomic classifier of metastatic risk on postoperative treatment recommendations for prostate cancer patients: a report from the DECIDE study group. Oncotarget. 2013;4(4):600–9.
51. Nguyen PL, Shin H, Yousefi K, et al. Impact of a genomic classifier of metastatic risk on post-prostatectomy treatment recommendations by radiation oncologists and urologists. Urology. 2015;86(1):35–40.
52. Swanson GP, Hussey MA, Tangen CM, et al. Predominant treatment failure in postprostatectomy patients is local: analysis of patterns of treatment failure in SWOG 8794. J Clin Oncol. 2007;25(16):2225–9.
53. Moinpour CM, Hayden KA, Unger JM, et al. Health-related quality of life results in pathologic stage C prostate cancer from a Southwest Oncology Group trial comparing radical prostatectomy alone with radical prostatectomy plus radiation therapy. J Clin Oncol. 2008;26(1):112–20.
54. Trock BJ, Han M, Freedland SJ, et al. Prostate cancer-specific survival following salvage radiotherapy vs observation in men with biochemical recurrence after radical prostatectomy. JAMA. 2008;299(23):2760–9.
55. Cotter SE, Chen MH, Moul JW, et al. Salvage radiation in men after prostate-specific antigen failure and the risk of death. Cancer. 2011;117(17):3925–32.
56. Stephenson AJ, Scardino PT, Kattan MW, et al. Predicting the outcome of salvage radiation therapy for recurrent prostate cancer after radical prostatectomy. J Clin Oncol. 2007;25(15):2035–41.
57. Tendulkar RD, Agrawal S, Gao T, et al. Contemporary update of a multi-institutional predictive nomogram for salvage radiotherapy after radical prostatectomy. J Clin Oncol. 2016.
58. Abugharib A, Jackson WC, Tumati V, et al. Very early salvage radiotherapy improves distant metastasis-free survival. J Urol. 2017;197(3 Pt 1):662–8.
59. Stish BJ, Pisansky TM, Harmsen WS, et al. Improved metastasis-free and survival outcomes with early salvage radiotherapy in men with detectable prostate-specific antigen after prostatectomy for prostate cancer. J Clin Oncol. 2016;34(32):3864–71.
60. Parker C, Sydes MR, Catton C, et al. Radiotherapy and androgen deprivation in combination after local surgery (RADICALS): a new Medical Research Council/National Cancer Institute of Canada phase III trial of adjuvant treatment after radical prostatectomy. BJU Int. 2007;99(6):1376–9.
61. Pearse M, Fraser-Browne C, Davis ID, et al. A phase III trial to investigate the timing of radiotherapy for prostate cancer with high-risk features: background and rationale of the radiotherapy—adjuvant versus early salvage (RAVES) trial. BJU Int. 2014;113(Suppl 2):7–12.
62. Richaud P, Sargos P, Henriques de Figueiredo B, et al. Postoperative radiotherapy of prostate cancer. Cancer Radiotherapie. 2010;14(6–7):500–3.
63. Shipley WU, Seiferheld W, Lukka HR, et al. Radiation with or without Antiandrogen therapy in recurrent prostate cancer. N Engl J Med. 2017;376(5):417–28.
64. Carrie C, Hasbini A, de Laroche G, et al. Salvage radiotherapy with or without short-term hormone therapy for rising prostate-specific antigen concentration after radical prostatec-

tomy (GETUG-AFU 16): a randomised, multicentre, open-label phase 3 trial. Lancet Oncol. 2016;17(6):747–56.
65. Jackson WC, Schipper MJ, Johnson SB, et al. Duration of androgen deprivation therapy influences outcomes for patients receiving radiation therapy following radical prostatectomy. Eur Urol. 2016;69(1):50–7.
66. Hurwitz MD, Harris J, Sartor O, et al. Adjuvant radiation therapy, androgen deprivation, and docetaxel for high-risk prostate cancer postprostatectomy: results of NRG Oncology/RTOG study 0621. Cancer. 2017;123(13):2489–96.
67. Perera M, Papa N, Christidis D, et al. Sensitivity, specificity, and predictors of positive 68Ga-prostate-specific membrane antigen positron emission tomography in advanced prostate cancer: a systematic review and meta-analysis. Eur Urol. 2016;70(6):926–37.
68. Zhao SG, Chang SL, Spratt DE, et al. Development and validation of a 24-gene predictor of response to postoperative radiotherapy in prostate cancer: a matched, retrospective analysis. Lancet Oncol. 2016;17(11):1612–20.
69. Den RB, Yousefi K, Trabulsi EJ, et al. Genomic classifier identifies men with adverse pathology after radical prostatectomy who benefit from adjuvant radiation therapy. J Clin Oncol. 2015;33(8):944–51.
70. Zhao SG, Chang SL, Erho N, et al. Associations of luminal and basal subtyping of prostate cancer with prognosis and response to androgen deprivation therapy. JAMA Oncol. 2017;3(12):1663–72.

Chapter 8
Biochemical Recurrence After Radiation Therapy

Christopher Martin and William Lowrance

Clinical Case Scenario: Three years after receiving proton beam therapy for treatment of low volume, Gleason score 7 (3 + 4) (grade group 3) prostate cancer with a PSA value of 8.6 ng/mL, a healthy 68-year-old man wants to discuss his best management options His posttreatment nadir was 0.8 ng/mL, 12 months after treatment. Since then it has continued to rise with 1.4 ng/mL at 1½ years, 2.2 ng/mL at 2 years, 3.3 ng/mL at 2½ years, and most recently 4.5 ng/mL at 3 years. Metastatic survey (CT abdomen and pelvis, bone scan) is negative, and he wants to discuss management and treatment options.

This patient in this scenario is considered intermediate risk category based on NCCN criteria [1]. Although he received proton beam therapy for his radiation, he was also eligible for photon-based external beam radiation therapy (EBRT) as well as high- and low-dose brachytherapy [1]. Proton-based therapy differs in mechanism from photon-based radiation in respect to the distance the energy form can travel [2]. Theoretically, due to the larger mass of the proton, the distance of travel beyond the prostate would be decreased, thus reducing the risk of radiation exposure to other organs [2]. While arguments will continue to be made regarding the oncologic outcomes and side effects of primary treatment, there is no evidence that evaluation and treatment of biochemical recurrence should meaningfully differ between proton- and photon-based therapies. Thus this chapter will cover biochemical recurrence after all of the radiation therapies and will include the nuances of evaluation and treatment where evidence exists.

C. Martin, B.S. (✉) · W. Lowrance, M.D., M.P.H.
Division of Urology, Department of Surgery, Huntsman Cancer Institute, University of Utah, Salt Lake City, UT, USA
e-mail: Christopher.martin@hci.utah.edu; Will.Lowrance@hci.utah.edu

© Springer International Publishing AG, part of Springer Nature 2018   101
S. S. Chang, M. S. Cookson (eds.), *Prostate Cancer*,
https://doi.org/10.1007/978-3-319-78646-9_8

Screening/Surveillance

Recurrence Risk

After definitive therapy for prostate cancer, a primary consideration is a recurrence risk and cancer-specific mortality. Overall, approximately 33% of patients will have a biochemical failure after definitive radiation therapy [3]. The important determinants of this risk are the type of radiation therapy used, the presence of concurrent hormone therapy, PSA kinetics (velocity, density, posttreatment nadir, and other subcomponents), and most importantly the extent of disease at time of treatment (as determined by clinical stage, Gleason score, and PSA value) [4, 5]. Modern-day radiation techniques utilize higher doses of radiation that have improved cancer-specific outcomes compared to lower doses used in the past [5]. This also appears to be the case with proton-based therapies, with higher doses significantly reducing the biochemical recurrence rates [6]. While some studies have suggested proton-based therapies have a lower risk of recurrence, these risks appear equivalent when stratified by risk group [7].

Concurrent Androgen Deprivation Therapy

Multiple phase III clinical trials have consistently demonstrated that concurrent hormonal therapy with radiation therapy lowers the risk of recurrence and metastasis [8–15]. This benefit is most apparent in patients with high and intermediate risk prostate cancer. The patient from this clinical scenario initially had NCCN intermediate risk disease and could have been offered, and many would say, should have been offered, concurrent androgen deprivation therapy (ADT) with his radiation. In patients with low-risk disease, the evidence supporting concomitant utilization of ADT with radiation therapy is less robust.

PSA Kinetics

Three postradiation PSA variables have been associated with risk of biochemical recurrence (BCR): PSA nadir, time to nadir, and PSA doubling time. Value of the PSA nadir is an independent predictor of biochemical control of prostate cancer, with patients who achieve a ≤ 0.5 ng/mL nadir (without ADT) and will have 5-year BCR-free survival rates of 90% [16]. There does not appear to be a lower limit to this relationship; the lower the nadir value, the lower the patient's risk [17]. In fact, some models suggest that posttreatment nadir is a stronger predictor of biochemical recurrence than pretreatment PSA [18].

Another PSA-specific factor associated with BCR is the time to PSA nadir. Increased nadir times are associated with improved rates of BCR-free survival, with one series showing that 6, 12, 24, and >24 months to PSA nadir had a 27, 32, 42, and 74% rate of disease-free survival [19]. The last and potentially most important PSA-specific factor is the PSA doubling time after treatment. Patients with a doubling time of <6 months had a metastatic-free survival of 50% compared to 83% for those with a doubling time of >6 months [20]. Much like with the nadir value, there has not been an established threshold for doubling time consistently associated with a specific clinical outcome. In general, longer PSA doubling times are associated with improved oncologic outcomes.

Disease-Specific Risk

The Gleason score or grade group is highly predictive of biochemical and disease-specific recurrence and is typically considered to carry the most prognostic value of any clinical variable [21]. The other cancer-specific variables that impact disease recurrence are the estimated volume of disease and PSA velocity or doubling time, but overall disease burden can be difficult to measure without a surgical specimen, and its specific impact after radiation treatment is poorly characterized [22, 23].

Surveillance Schedule

An initial clinical decision point after definitive therapy is the surveillance schedule for PSA testing as well as the type of PSA test. While PSA surveillance testing in prostate cancer patients post treatment is considerably more sensitive and specific than PSA screening in the general population, little evidence-based guidance exists on the optimal surveillance intervals. NCCN guidelines suggest PSA be monitored every 6–12 months after treatment for the first 5 years and annually thereafter [1]. Some data suggest that surveillance PSA testing after radical prostatectomy can be discontinued after 10 years in men with undetectable PSA values [24]. However, no such evidence has been presented for patients treated with radiation therapy. AUA, ASTRO, and SUO guidelines suggest frequency be determined by risk of relapse and patient preferences [25]. While ultrasensitive PSA testing (measuring PSA to the hundredth decimal position) has potential to change management in postprostatectomy patients, the higher biochemical threshold and average PSA values in patients treated with radiation likely make this test less useful in the postradiation setting. Standard PSA testing (measuring PSA to the one tenth decimal) seems adequately sensitive for the determination of BCR after radiation.

Diagnosis

The purpose of following patients' PSA values after definitive therapy is to identify recurrence of prostate cancer. However, the actual threshold of what constitutes recurrence after radiation therapy in an individual patient is not entirely standardized or understood.

Variation Between Radiation and Surgery

Benign Prostate Tissue

One of the most important differences in diagnosis of biochemical recurrence (BCR) of prostate cancer after radiation therapy compared to surgery is the likelihood of remaining benign prostate tissue [26]. After adequate treatment of prostate cancer with radical prostatectomy, there should be no viable prostate tissue (benign or cancerous), and the value of PSA should drop to zero and thus leave a very low threshold for biochemical recurrence. By contrast in radiation therapy, benign tissue is often retained within the prostate and the threshold in which to determine biochemical failure is much less precise. In fact, even cancerous tissue can continue to undergo apoptosis for up to 30 months after treatment [26, 27]. Because of this the values of PSA in patients cured with radiation therapy can vary, and many of the values considered as the threshold for biochemical recurrence only give a relative likelihood of clinical recurrence or progression.

PSA Bounce

The difficulty in establishing a diagnosis of recurrence is further increased by the potential for continued tumor apoptosis after treatment as well as the potential for a PSA bounce [28]. In patients adequately treated with radical prostatectomy shortly after surgery, PSA reaches its nadir quickly; with a half-life of 2–3 days, a patient's PSA should be undetectable within 4–6 weeks post prostatectomy [29]. Thus, significant elevations after radical prostatectomy should be considered malignant in nature or the result of an incomplete gland resection.

Comparatively, in patients treated with radiation, this pattern is more sporadic [30]. Postradiation death of tumor cells can continue well over a year after treatment, and the PSA value can take 18–36 months to reach its nadir [26]. Over this time period, the PSA value can have an acute elevation that is commonly referred to as a bounce [30]. Although more common in brachytherapy, this pattern has been found in external beam patients as well and can occur 1–2 years after treatment and last for up to 8 months [31].

This bounce phenomenon further complicates follow-up and can be mistaken for recurrence or disease progression. It is unclear whether this is an inflammatory or immunological response to tumor, prostatitis, or some other factor, but the immunological hypothesis has the most evidence [32]. The presence of a bounce has been suggested as a positive prognostic factor in some studies [33]. However, this finding has been questioned and further evaluation is necessary [31].

Biochemical Recurrence Definition

Historical/Alternative Criteria

In 1996 American Society for Radiation Oncology (ASTRO) criteria defined biochemical failure as three consecutive rises in PSA value after a nadir with the date of failure set as halfway between the date of the third rise and the date of the nadir value [34]. This definition did not correlate to clinical progression or survival and did not identify recurrence accurately in patients undergoing hormonal therapy, and the date of failure using backdating made Kaplan-Meier estimates of recurrence-free survival inaccurate. Additionally, this criterion was very susceptible to false positives resulting from PSA bounce [35]. Prior to development of updated criteria in 2005, around 70 variations of the 1996 ASTRO criteria and more than 99 definitions overall had been published regarding biochemical recurrence [36]. As such, standardization among the diagnosis was sorely needed.

Phoenix Criteria

The initial ASTRO criteria performed poorly in patients on concurrent hormonal therapy and other clinical scenarios. ASTRO then created the Phoenix criteria defined as a 2 ng/mL rise above the nadir (with or without concurrent hormonal therapy) with date of failure based on the date of the 2 ng/mL rise [37]. Studies comparing the criteria show that Phoenix criteria have a lower false-positive rate but are vulnerable to isolated PSA rises [38]. With this issue in mind, there is an imbalance between the false positives associated with an acute PSA bounce and a potential to miss the window of localized recurrence. Regardless of its shortcomings, the Phoenix criteria appear to be more accurate in diagnosis of clinically meaningful BCR as compared to the ASTRO criteria [39, 40]. Based on these criteria, our patient definitively meets the definition of BCR after radiation therapy and very likely has some type of recurrence, and salvage therapy can be considered.

Evaluation

Sites of Recurrence

In men diagnosed with a BCR, 60–70% will have biopsy-confirmed prostatic disease. This slightly varies in men with clinically detected recurrence, and their recurrence pattern is as follows: 55% local, 33% bone, 21% pelvic nodes, and 9% abdominal nodes. Though there appears to be a high rate of localized disease, current imaging modalities are not adequately accurate to exclude the possibility of missed metastatic disease or micrometastatic disease, and as such, localized therapy can often be attempted in patients with unidentified extraprostatic cancer. Though this risk is always present, a thorough evaluation can help mitigate some of these risks.

Traditional Evaluation

Imaging Evaluation

The AUA, NCCN, and EUA do not have definitive recommendations for imaging in the setting of biochemical recurrence. However, guidelines do state that imaging in the setting of biochemical recurrence should only be pursued when local or systemic therapy is being considered (Table 8.1). In patients uninterested in or poor candidates for localized therapy, imaging studies should only be pursued when PSA values or kinetics make risk of metastasis likely. Likewise, imaging should only be pursued in patients considering systemic therapy. The traditional imaging evaluation in patients with suspected recurrence in prostate cancer is a combination of bone imaging (often done with ^{99m}Tc-MDP) as well as CT or MRI. As each of these imaging modalities is prone to potential inaccuracies, it is important to pair imaging with other clinical parameters.

Bone Imaging

In the pretreatment phase, the PSA threshold for bone scan is typically 20 ng/mL unless other high-risk features are present (e.g., Gleason score ≥ 8). In the posttreatment phase, a bone scan is unlikely to be positive when the PSA is ≤5 ng/mL or the PSA doubling time is ≥10 months [41]. An issue with bone scans is the high rate of equivocal scans. Often regions of interest cannot be differentiated from reactive bone formation, and as such, findings may require follow-up over time. For patients being considered for definitive local salvage therapy, this strategy can often cause

Table 8.1 Evaluation of prostate cancer patients after radiation

Modality	Description	Advantage	Disadvantage	Contraindication/appropriate usage
CT	Computed tomographic imaging uses radiation along axial lines and computer programming to generate full images	High-quality scan, excellent at finding metastatic foci within solid organs	Radiation exposure, CT has particular difficulty identifying abnormalities in the prostate itself	Contrast should not be used in patients with limited renal capacity; scans should only be performed in patients considered for treatment
MRI	Magnetic resonance imaging allowing characterization of the prostate, nodes, and potential sites of metastasis	Recent improvements in MRI quality have improved the sensitivity of MRI for nodal disease, no radiation exposure	Presence of lymph node does not mean that tumor is present, and absence of findings does not exclude disease and thus often presents diagnostic dilemma and requires a time interval for correlation	Contrast should not be used in patients with limited renal capacity; scans should only be performed in patients considered for treatment
Bone scan	Technetium 99 bone scintigraphy	Low radiation dose can be used in patients with poor renal function	Accumulates in response to tumor and, however, also accumulates in degenerative joint disease, benign fractures, and inflammation	Likely unhelpful in patients with PSA <5 after definitive treatment with radiation
Biopsy	Targeting biopsy of the prostate (TRUS), lymph nodes, or potential metastatic site	Positive result allows definitive diagnosis of recurrence and on regional or metastatic survey allows avoidance of ineffective local therapy	Potential for false-negative results, difficulty associated with pathologic examination of radiated prostate	Should only be considered if pathological result will significantly change management

patients to miss the window of opportunity to treat a localized disease recurrence. One strategy shown to improve the accuracy of bone scans is the utilization of single-photon emission computerized tomography (SPECT) [42]. This imaging modality can be used on specific areas of interest such as the spine or instead used as whole-body SPECT.

CT Scan/MRI

Though the accuracy of MRI and CT scans has not been adequately evaluated in the recurrent prostate cancer setting, they have been well studied prior to initial treatment. The prevailing issue with both imaging modalities is the inability to detect small foci of cancer in lymph nodes as these imaging modalities have little ability to determine malignant from reactive changes in lymph nodes <1 cm. In larger lymph nodes, these imaging modalities have improved accuracy and also can be paired with fine needle aspiration or biopsy to improve further detection specificity [43].

Role of Biopsy

In patients with BCR who have imaging and PSA values suggesting localized disease, further workup is often necessary prior to treatment. Patients with biochemical recurrence after radical prostatectomy often do not need biopsies prior to salvage therapies. However, as discussed, the limitations with BCR diagnostic criteria after radiation make many diagnoses of recurrence more difficult to verify and localize. In patients with a borderline or moderate biochemical recurrence, especially when salvage prostatectomy is being considered, a TRUS biopsy for pathologic evidence of disease must be done. However the interpretation of pathologic prostate specimens after radiation treatment is difficult and requires an expert in prostate cancer pathology [44].

Emerging/Advanced Imaging

PET imaging will likely play a major role in the future diagnosis and differentiation of biochemically recurrent prostate cancer. Utilizing prostate-specific markers, PET imaging hopes to drastically improve the specificity and sensitivity for prostate tissue activity [45]. The issue with PET imaging in today's practice is the myriad of options, lack of standardization, and the lack of validated cutoffs for each individual radiotracer. The literature is filled with studies testing the emerging radionucleotides: 18F-fluorodeoxyglucose, 18F-choline, 18F-fluciclovine, 18F-FDHT, 11C-acetate, and 11C-choline. These radiotracers target prostate cancer tissue via various mechanisms such as glucose metabolism, lipogenesis, DNA synthesis, amino acid metabolism, androgen receptors, and even prostate-specific membrane antigens. The 18F-NaF PET also appears to improve on traditional bone scans [46]. While it is too early in their utilization to label one PET radiotracer superior, many of these PET imaging techniques appear to have superior sensitivity and specificity to traditional imaging modalities [45, 47]. These novel PET scans are not only improving the speed with which patients' recurrences can be identified through imaging, but they are also creating difficult clinical situations. These scans can often detect specific areas of likely recurrence at relatively low PSA values and potentially below the threshold for a PSA-based biochemical recurrence. For example, in patients with a single PET-avid lymph node, what relative roles should definitive local treatment, systemic treatment, or observation play in the clinical decision-making surrounding their care? While PET scans offer us the potential for significantly improved detection of recurrence, we may be receiving more information than we have clinical evidence to act upon.

Therapeutic Management

Localized Salvage Treatment

Considerations

Randomized trials comparing the salvage therapy options are lacking. In patients treated with radical prostatectomy, the primary salvage treatment option studied has been salvage radiation, and this appears to show a significant cancer-specific mortality benefit on retrospective series (Table 8.2). However, data on salvage therapies after definitive radiation therapy are heterogeneous and do not illustrate comparative efficacy [48, 49]. The paucity of evidence is illustrated in the remarkably low rate of local salvage therapy attempted with BCR after primary radiation therapy (as low as 2% in some series) [50]. It is unclear if this is due to a concern about treatment-related side effects, a belief that local salvage therapy lacks benefit, or if there is uncertainty surrounding the accurate identification of BCR in the early stages after radiation treatment and the ability to exclude the presence of systemic disease. It could also be that patients receiving radiation therapy for prostate cancer are on average older and their estimated life expectancy may prevent a benefit from local salvage therapy.

With these factors in mind, the most important task for a clinician is adequately assessing the location of the recurrence (local vs. distant) as local salvage treatments each have significant side effects and may have limited efficacy in altering the course of the disease when distant spread has already occurred. When considering a patient for local salvage therapy after RT failure, patients typically have a PSA value of <10 ng/mL, life expectancy of >10 years, a negative metastatic workup, and a full understanding of the possible treatment side effects.

Observation

The diagnosis of a biochemical recurrence does not necessarily mean that the patient will die from their prostate cancer [51]. Factors predictive of progression are a higher Gleason score, longer PSA doubling time, and longer time from treatment to BCR [23, 52]. Many patients do well with observation. For example, after radical

Table 8.2 Therapeutic management

Treatment	Description	Advantages	Disadvantages	Contraindications
Observation/ expectant management	Observation of patient until PSA or PSA doubling time passes a threshold making metastasis or progression likely or symptoms develop Followed by ADT	Avoids local salvage therapies and negative side effects in the short term Additionally for those that do not progress, they avoid intervention entirely	Not curative. For young (or those with long life expectancy) patients that can be cured locally, salvage treatments could offer improved quality of life	
Salvage prostatectomy	Surgical removal of prostate	For disease located within the prostate, likely represents highest chance for oncologic control	Morbid, worsened patient-reported outcomes, technically difficult procedure	Patients with limited life expectancy or who cannot tolerate procedure or anesthesia
Salvage radiation	Either repeated EBRT or brachytherapy	EBRT avoid requirement for anesthesia	Second round of radiation associated with significantly more complications	Severe or debilitating lower urinary tract symptoms. Prior transurethral resection of the prostate
Salvage cryotherapy	Freezing of prostate via percutaneous approach	Questionably less morbid than surgery, can be performed without general anesthesia	Likely represents poorer oncologic efficacy Incontinence, sexual dysfunction, and pain still an issue	Seminal vesicle involvement, prior treatment with ADT (relative)
Salvage HIFU	Thermal damage to prostate tissue via ultrasonic waves	Allows potential for unilateral salvage therapy	Appears to have lower oncologic efficacy	Large prostate (>50 cm^3) or prostatic calcification

prostatectomy, a man with Gleason <8, doubling time of >15 months, and >3 years from treatment to biochemical recurrence has an estimated 15-year cancer-specific mortality of only 6% [53]. Studies in patients treated with radiation therapy show similar outcomes, with 88% of patients free from disease metastasis 5 years after BCR [52]. Even after the development of metastasis, there is a median 5-year survival [54]. With salvage treatment options having a high associated morbidity and poor-quality data measuring efficacy, observation should be discussed as a possible treatment option in patients with favorable disease characteristics (prolonged PSA doubling time) or limited life expectancy.

Salvage Prostatectomy

Of the local treatments for biochemical recurrence after radiation therapy, salvage prostatectomy is the most extensively studied [55, 56]. Salvage radical prostatectomy after radiation is a more difficult procedure with worse oncologic and functional outcomes compared to primary radical prostatectomy [57, 58]. Among potent patients treated with salvage prostatectomy less than a quarter will be able to regain meaningful erectile function [57]. The rates of fistula, bladder neck contracture, rectal injury, and infection are also higher among patients undergoing salvage prostatectomy with a risk of rectal injury 4–9%, bladder neck contracture 14–18%, and incontinence (requiring pads) in 30–41% [57–59]. Although salvage radical prostatectomy appears to lower the risk of BCR (slightly less than 50% BCR-free at 10 years), metastasis, and prostate-specific mortality, such trials are not randomized and have not adequately compared overall mortality between surgery, other salvage options, and expectant management [49, 60, 61]. There are two other important caveats to these studies. First, when comparing the biochemical failure rates between salvage therapy options, diagnosis of post-prostatectomy BCR compared to BCR after other salvage treatments is likely much more sensitive due to the lower PSA threshold [62]. Thus, local recurrence, micrometastatic, and oligometastatic disease has a higher likelihood of going unrecognized in the other salvage treatment options. When looking at disease progression and response rates, it is also important to realize that trials involving prostatectomy could have healthier patients than those that utilize other treatment modalities. Thus to have definitive evidence, randomized trials between salvage treatment options are necessary with overall mortality and disease-specific mortality as more important endpoints for salvage therapies than BCR. Given the available evidence, patients appropriate for salvage prostatectomy are those men that are relatively healthy, having a > 10-year life expectancy, have local recurrence only, have good baseline urinary function, and have been adequately counseled on the increased risks of incontinence and impotence associated with the procedure [61]. Our patient meets this criterion, and salvage prostatectomy can be considered in this patient.

Salvage Radiation

Another option when a patient has a local recurrence of prostate cancer after radiation therapy is salvage local radiation therapy. The most extensively studied of these options after EBRT is salvage brachytherapy. This has moderate oncologic efficacy with some series suggesting 88% of patients BCR-free at 3 years of follow-up [63, 64]. However, this value decreases to closer to 20–50% at 5-year follow-up [64, 65]. An important benefit to this treatment option is the ability to perform salvage treatment in patients with severe comorbidities or those who would not undergo prostatectomy. However, those patients are also less likely to benefit from such treatments as with each increase in competing risk factors for overall mortality, the likelihood of dying of prostate cancer decreases. The rates of complications after brachytherapy are elevated with increased risks of urinary and gastrointestinal complications [64]. Another issue is brachytherapy and is difficult to accomplish in patients that have had a prior transurethral resection of the prostate or in those who have prostate volumes >60–70 cm^3. Salvage EBRT is also an option with series suggesting about half of patients are BCR-free at 2 years of follow-up [66]. However, much like brachytherapy, the associated side effects are more pronounced in the salvage setting than in the primary treatment setting.

Salvage Cryoablation

Cryoablation of the prostate after radiation treatment is another local salvage therapy option. With most cryotherapy treatments, there will be a rim of periurethral prostate tissue preserved, and as such PSA values are not expected to nadir as low as prostatectomy levels [67]. This zone of untreated tissue makes patients with seminal vesicle involvement poor candidates for cryoablation. The presence of untreated tissue also leads to confusion about the posttreatment PSA levels, and many studies chose to use Phoenix, ASTRO, or a unique set of criteria for diagnosis of posttreatment biochemical failure. This makes comparing trials difficult. Early oncologic data on cryosurgery is favorable with up to 78% BCR-free survival at 7 years based on a biochemical threshold of 1.0 ng/mL [68]. However, these results can be quite variable with one of the largest trials to date published more recently having a 34% rate of biochemical recurrence-free survival for patients at little over 3 years of follow-up [69]. Treatment with cryoablation also comes with severe potential side effects such as rectal and urethral injuries. This risk decreased with the newer gas-based cryoablation technology with improved continence rates and rate of rectal fistulas dropping to >1% [70]. However, the negative effects on erectile function have not improved with rates of impotence hovering around 90%. Though some trials have shown promise with using hemiablation of the prostate to lower the morbidity of the procedure without affecting oncologic control, caution should be applied to the possibility of multifocal recurrence [71]. Additionally, studies suggest that the optimal patient for salvage cryotherapy has a PSA doubling time of >16 months, as a doubling time less than this value has been associated with biochemical recurrence [72]. Unfortunately many patients with a doubling time that prolonged have a low risk of prostate-specific mortality and might not benefit from localized salvage treatment and would almost certainly lose their erectile function. For study comparisons to be valid, there needs to be consistency in the definition of biochemical recurrence, or definitive diagnoses should be confirmed via pretreatment and posttreatment tissue sampling.

Salvage HIFU

Limited studies have looked at high-intensity focused ultrasound (HIFU) for localized recurrence of prostate cancer treated with radiotherapy. The main issue with comparison between the treatment types is the percentage of patients treated that would be considered high risk. This severely limits the comparative value of the studies. After previous failures to acquire approval, the FDA has recently approved HIFU for ablation of prostate tissue, but this term is not specific for prostate cancer. However, it appears that HIFU treatment has efficacy in treatment of localized prostate cancer recurrences, especially in low-risk patients [73–75]. HIFU even appears to be a potential option for focal therapy in patients with highly localized recurrences [76]. Much like the other salvage treatments, low PSA nadir after HIFU is a strongly positive prognostic factor [77]. However, this treatment appears to be a poor treatment option for those with high-risk disease with BCR-free estimates of less than a third of patients at 3 years of follow-up [73]. HIFU also appears to be a poor treatment option for patients with cancer recurrence located anterior to the urethra [78]. Furthermore, for patients requiring a biopsy after undergoing salvage HIFU, there are significant challenges to pathological interpretation making further treatment planning difficult [79]. Compared to primary HIFU, there is a significantly elevated risk of urinary retention, urinary incontinence (often requiring an intervention such as artificial urinary sphincter implantation), erectile dysfunction, and urethral fistula [75, 80]. However, despite these increased risks, it appears that HIFU still represents a local salvage therapy treatment option, but the quality of evidence supporting it is the lowest among the local treatment modalities [81].

Distant Salvage Treatment

Treatment of Oligometastatic Disease with Radiation or Surgical Excision

There is expanding interest in the treatment of prostate cancer recurrence in the setting of oligometastatic disease with some type of local therapy. The important issue here is weighing the small potential for curative therapy and the likely potential for delaying ADT against the potential for treatment complications. Many of these clinical decisions have emerged as imaging modalities such as PET scans have allowed more accurate identification of cancerous prostate tissue throughout the body [45]. Radiation treatment of metastatic foci appears to prolong progression-free survival (PFS) with patients having a PFS of 1–3 years after radiation treatment [82–84]. However, when interpreting relative efficacy of treatments for oligometastatic disease, it is important to understand that such patients already have a > 6-year median life expectancy and many patients in these studies are included despite concomitant ADT use [82]. While these trials have high recurrence rates, they show that treatment of oligometastatic disease can potentially delay eventual treatment with ADT [85, 86]. Given the significant side effects of ADT, these treatments have the potential to improve patients' quality of life [87].

Systemic Treatment Options

Androgen Deprivation Therapy

For symptomatic disease recurrence or clinically detected metastases on imaging, ADT should be considered, especially in hormone-naive patients. In men treated expectantly with ADT for metastasis, many will live >15 years [87].

Conclusion

Our patient was considered intermediate risk status prior to his original treatment. At this point he has experienced a biochemical failure and has a very strong potential for disease recurrence. With a PSA of 4.5, metastasis is less likely, but imaging modalities are not adequately sensitive to eliminate the possibility of metastatic foci. At this point we have a very healthy gentleman with what appears to be local recurrence of previously intermediate risk prostate cancer. Without any treatment, this recurrence has the potential to metastasize and cause morbidity and even mortality in this patient. We recommend discussing the local salvage therapy options. We might recommend salvage radical prostatectomy in this case, ensuring the patient has a good understanding that the procedure has a significant risk of altering his quality of life and that these risks are elevated above the typical patient undergoing primary radical prostatectomy. If the patient selects this treatment option, we would recommend both a TRUS biopsy to confirm local disease and a fluciclovine PET scan to increase our confidence in the presence of both local recurrence and absence of nodal disease or metastasis. Other local salvage therapies are certainly options as well. The patient could also consider a watchful waiting approach with plans to initiate ADT at the time of detection of clinical metastasis. Note that ongoing studies will soon further our understanding of the role of newer ADT modalities in the BCR setting.

References

1. Mohler JL, Armstrong AJ, Bahnson RR, et al. Prostate cancer, version 1.2016. J Natl Compr Cancer Netw. 2016;14:19.
2. Wisenbaugh ES, Andrews PE, Ferrigni RG, et al. Proton beam therapy for localized prostate cancer 101: basics, controversies, and facts. Rev Urol. 2014;16:67.

3. Kuban DA, Thames HD, Levy LB, et al. Long-term multi-institutional analysis of stage T1–T2 prostate cancer treated with radiotherapy in the PSA era. Int J Radiat Oncol Biol Phys. 2003;57:915.
4. Kattan MW, Zelefsky MJ, Kupelian PA, et al. Pretreatment Nomogram for predicting the outcome of three-dimensional conformal radiotherapy in prostate cancer. J Clin Oncol. 2000;18:3352.
5. Zietman AL, DeSilvio ML, Slater JD, et al. Comparison of conventional-dose vs high-dose conformal radiation therapy in clinically localized adenocarcinoma of the prostate: a randomized controlled trial. JAMA. 2005;294:1233.
6. Zietman AL, Bae K, Slater JD, et al. Randomized trial comparing conventional-dose with high-dose conformal radiation therapy in early-stage adenocarcinoma of the prostate: long-term results from proton radiation oncology group/american college of radiology 95-09. J Clin Oncol. 2010;28:1106.
7. Coen JJ, Zietman AL, Rossi CJ, et al. Comparison of high-dose proton radiotherapy and brachytherapy in localized prostate cancer: a case-matched analysis. Int J Radiat Oncol Biol Phys. 2012;82:e25.
8. Bolla M, Collette L, Blank L, et al. Long-term results with immediate androgen suppression and external irradiation in patients with locally advanced prostate cancer (an EORTC study): a phase III randomised trial. Lancet. 2002;360:103.
9. Widmark A, Klepp O, Solberg A, et al. Endocrine treatment, with or without radiotherapy, in locally advanced prostate cancer (SPCG-7/SFUO-3): an open randomised phase III trial. Lancet. 2009;373:301.
10. Tyrrell CJ, Payne H, See WA, et al. Bicalutamide ('Casodex') 150mg as adjuvant to radiotherapy in patients with localised or locally advanced prostate cancer: results from the randomised early prostate cancer Programme. Radiother Oncol. 2005;76:4.
11. Pilepich MV, Winter K, Lawton CA, et al. Androgen suppression adjuvant to definitive radiotherapy in prostate carcinoma—long-term results of phase III RTOG 85–31. Int J Radiat Oncol Biol Phys. 2005;61:1285.
12. Zagars GK, Johnson DE, von Eschenbach AC, et al. Adjuvant estrogen following radiation therapy for stage C adenocarcinoma of the prostate: long-term results of a prospective randomized study. Int J Radiat Oncol Biol Phys. 1988;14:1085.
13. D'Amico AV, Schultz D, Loffredo M, et al. Biochemical outcome following external beam radiation therapy with or without androgen suppression therapy for clinically localized prostate cancer. JAMA. 2000;284:1280.
14. Jones CU, Hunt D, McGowan DG, et al. Radiotherapy and short-term androgen deprivation for localized prostate cancer. N Engl J Med. 2011;365:107.
15. D'Amico AV, Manola J, Loffredo M, et al. 6-month androgen suppression plus radiation therapy vs radiation therapy alone for patients with clinically localized prostate cancer: a randomized controlled trial. JAMA. 2004;292:821.
16. Zietman AL, Tibbs MK, Dallow KC, et al. Use of PSA nadir to predict subsequent biochemical outcome following external beam radiation therapy for T1-2 adenocarcinoma of the prostate. Radiother Oncol. 1996;40:159.
17. Critz FA, Williams WH, Holladay CT, et al. Post-treatment PSA ≤0.2 ng/ml defines disease freedom after radiotherapy for prostate cancer using modern techniques. Urology. 1999;54:968.
18. Crook JM, Bahadur YA, Bociek RG, et al. Radiotherapy for localized prostate carcinoma. The correlation of pretreatment prostate specific antigen and nadir prostate specific antigen with outcome as assessed by systematic biopsy and serum prostate specific antigen. Cancer. 1997;79:328.
19. Ray ME, Thames HD, Levy LB, et al. PSA nadir predicts biochemical and distant failures after external beam radiotherapy for prostate cancer: a multi-institutional analysis. Int J Radiat Oncol Biol Phys. 2006;64:1140.
20. Klayton TL, Ruth K, Buyyounouski MK, et al. PSA doubling time predicts for the development of distant metastases for patients who fail 3DCRT or IMRT using the phoenix definition. Pract Radiat Oncol. 2011;1:235.

21. Epstein JI, Egevad L, Amin MB, et al. The 2014 International Society of Urological Pathology (ISUP) consensus conference on Gleason grading of prostatic carcinoma: definition of grading patterns and proposal for a new grading system. Am J Surg Pathol. 2016;40:244.
22. D'Amico AV, Renshaw AA, Sussman B, et al. Pretreatment psa velocity and risk of death from prostate cancer following external beam radiation therapy. JAMA. 2005;294:440.
23. Lee AK, Levy LB, Cheung R, et al. Prostate-specific antigen doubling time predicts clinical outcome and survival in prostate cancer patients treated with combined radiation and hormone therapy. Int J Radiat Oncol Biol Phys. 2005;63:456.
24. Loeb S, Feng Z, Ross A, et al. Can we stop prostate specific antigen testing 10 years after radical prostatectomy? J Urol. 2012;186:500.
25. Sanda MG, et al. Clinically localized prostate cancer: AUA/ASTRO/SUO guideline. Part I: risk stratification, shared decision making, and care options. J Urol. 2017.
26. Crook JM, Perry GA, Robertson S, et al. Routine prostate biopsies following radiotherapy for prostate cancer: results for 226 patients. Urology. 1995;45:624.
27. Crook J, Malone S, Perry G, et al. Postradiotherapy prostate biopsies: what do they really mean? Results for 498 patients. Int J Radiat Oncol Biol Phys. 2000;48:355.
28. Zwahlen DR, Smith R, Andrianopoulos N, et al. Prostate-specific antigen bounce after permanent iodine-125 prostate brachytherapy—an Australian analysis. Int J Radiat Oncol Biol Phys. 2011;79:179.
29. Poyet C, Hof D, Sulser T, et al. Artificial prostate-specific antigen persistence after radical prostatectomy. J Clin Oncol. 2012;30:e62.
30. Rodriguez MA, Escutia MA, Antolin AR, et al. PSA bounce phenomenon after local treatment with radiation for prostate cancer. Arch Esp Urol. 2012;65:21.
31. Hanlon AL, Pinover WH, Horwitz EM, et al. Patterns and fate of PSA bouncing following 3D-CRT. Int J Radiat Oncol Biol Phys. 2001;50:845.
32. Yamamoto Y, Offord CP, Kimura G, et al. Tumour and immune cell dynamics explain the PSA bounce after prostate cancer brachytherapy. Br J Cancer. 2016;115:195.
33. Bernstein MB, Ohri N, Hodge JW, et al. Prostate-specific antigen bounce predicts for a favorable prognosis following brachytherapy: a meta-analysis. J Contemp Brachytherapy. 2013;5:210.
34. Consensus statement: guidelines for PSA following radiation therapy. American Society for Therapeutic Radiology and Oncology Consensus Panel. Int J Radiat Oncol Biol Phys. 1997;37:1035.
35. Zietman AL, Christodouleas JP, Shipley WU. PSA bounces after neoadjuvant androgen deprivation and external beam radiation: impact on definitions of failure. Int J Radiat Oncol Biol Phys. 2005;62:714.
36. Cookson MS, Aus G, Burnett AL, et al. Variation in the definition of biochemical recurrence in patients treated for localized prostate cancer: the American Urological Association prostate guidelines for localized prostate cancer update panel report and recommendations for a standard in the reporting of surgical outcomes. J Urol. 2007;177:540.
37. Roach M, Hanks G, Thames H, et al. Defining biochemical failure following radiotherapy with or without hormonal therapy in men with clinically localized prostate cancer: recommendations of the RTOG-ASTRO Phoenix Consensus Conference. Int J Radiat Oncol Biol Phys. 2006;65:965.
38. Denham JW, Kumar M, Gleeson PS, et al. Recognizing false biochemical failure calls after radiation with or without neo-adjuvant androgen deprivation for prostate cancer. Int J Radiat Oncol Biol Phys. 2009;74:404.
39. Horwitz EM, Thames HD, Kuban DA, et al. Definitions of biochemical failure that best predict clinical failure in patients with prostate cancer treated with external beam radiation alone: a multi-institutional pooled analysis. J Urol. 2005;173:797.
40. Abramowitz MC, Li T, Buyyounouski MK, et al. The Phoenix definition of biochemical failure predicts for overall survival in patients with prostate cancer. Cancer. 2008;112:55.
41. Choueiri TK, Dreicer R, Paciorek A, et al. A model that predicts the probability of positive imaging in prostate cancer cases with biochemical failure after initial definitive local therapy. J Urol. 2008;179:906.

42. Even-Sapir E, Metser U, Mishani E, et al. The detection of bone metastases in patients with high-risk prostate cancer: 99mTc-MDP planar bone scintigraphy, single- and multi-field-of-view SPECT, 18F-fluoride PET, and 18F-fluoride PET/CT. J Nucl Med. 2006;47:287.
43. Oyen RH, Van Poppel HP, Ameye FE, et al. Lymph node staging of localized prostatic carcinoma with CT and CT-guided fine-needle aspiration biopsy: prospective study of 285 patients. Radiology. 1994;190:315.
44. Molinie V, Mahjoub WK, Balaton A. Histological modifications observed in prostate after preserving treatments for prostate cancer and their impact on Gleason score interpretation. Ann Pathol. 2008;28:363.
45. Einspieler I, Rauscher I, Duwel C, et al. Detection efficacy of hybrid 68Ga-PSMA ligand PET/CT in prostate cancer patients with biochemical recurrence after primary radiation therapy defined by phoenix criteria. J Nucl Med. 2017;58:1081.
46. Segall GM. PET/CT with sodium 18F-fluoride for management of patients with prostate cancer. J Nucl Med. 2014;55:531.
47. Parker WP, Davis BJ, Park SS, et al. Identification of site-specific recurrence following primary radiation therapy for prostate cancer using C-11 choline positron emission tomography/computed tomography: a nomogram for predicting extrapelvic disease. Eur Urol. 2017;71:340.
48. Grossfeld GD, Stier DM, Flanders SC, et al. Use of second treatment following definitive local therapy for prostate cancer: data from the capsure database. J Urol. 1998;160:1398.
49. Peters M, Moman MR, van der Poel HG, et al. Patterns of outcome and toxicity after salvage prostatectomy, salvage cryosurgery and salvage brachytherapy for prostate cancer recurrences after radiation therapy: a multi-center experience and literature review. World J Urol. 2013;31:403.
50. Tran H, Kwok J, Pickles T, et al. Underutilization of local salvage therapy after radiation therapy for prostate cancer. Urol Oncol. 2014;32:701.
51. Faria SL, Mahmud S, Souhami L, et al. No immediate treatment after biochemical failure in patients with prostate cancer treated by external beam radiotherapy. Urology. 2006;67:142.
52. Pinover WH, Horwitz EM, Hanlon AL, et al. Validation of a treatment policy for patients with prostate specific antigen failure after three-dimensional conformal prostate radiation therapy. Cancer. 2003;97:1127.
53. Freedland SJ, Humphreys EB, Mangold LA, et al. Risk of prostate cancer-specific mortality following biochemical recurrence after radical prostatectomy. JAMA. 2005;294:433.
54. Pound CR, Partin AW, Eisenberger MA, et al. Natural history of progression after psa elevation following radical prostatectomy. JAMA. 1999;281:1591.
55. Chade DC, Eastham J, Graefen M, et al. Cancer control and functional outcomes of salvage radical prostatectomy for radiation-recurrent prostate cancer: a systematic review of the literature. Eur Urol. 2012;61:961.
56. Pisters LL, Leibovici D, Blute M, et al. Locally recurrent prostate cancer after initial radiation therapy: a comparison of salvage radical prostatectomy versus cryotherapy. J Urol. 2009;182:517.
57. Gotto GT, Yunis LH, Vora K, et al. Impact of prior prostate radiation on complications after radical prostatectomy. J Urol. 2010;184:136.
58. Bates AS, Samavedi S, Kumar A, et al. Salvage robot assisted radical prostatectomy: a propensity matched study of perioperative, oncological and functional outcomes. Eur J Surg Oncol. 2015;41:1540.
59. Nguyen PL, D'Amico AV, Lee AK, et al. Patient selection, cancer control, and complications after salvage local therapy for postradiation prostate-specific antigen failure: a systematic review of the literature. Cancer. 2007;110:1417.
60. Chade DC, Shariat SF, Cronin AM, et al. Salvage radical prostatectomy for radiation-recurrent prostate cancer: a multi-institutional collaboration. Eur Urol. 2011;60:205.
61. Touma NJ, Izawa JI, Chin JL. Current status of local salvage therapies following radiation failure for prostate cancer. J Urol. 2005;173:373.
62. Xia J, Trock BJ, Gulati R, et al. Overdetection of recurrence after radical prostatectomy: estimates based on patient and tumor characteristics. Clin Cancer Res. 2014;20:5302.

63. Peters M, Maenhout M, van der Voort van Zyp JR, et al. Focal salvage iodine-125 brachyther-apy for prostate cancer recurrences after primary radiotherapy: a retrospective study regarding toxicity, biochemical outcome and quality of life. Radiother Oncol. 2014;112:77.
64. Yamada Y, Okihara K, Iwata T, et al. Salvage brachytherapy for locally recurrent prostate can-cer after external beam radiotherapy. Asian J Androl. 2015;17:899.
65. Chen CP, Weinberg V, Shinohara K, et al. Salvage HDR brachytherapy for recurrent prostate cancer after previous definitive radiation therapy: 5-year outcomes. Int J Radiat Oncol Biol Phys. 2013;86:324.
66. Zerini D, Jereczek-Fossa BA, Fodor C, et al. Salvage image-guided intensity modu-lated or stereotactic body reirradiation of local recurrence of prostate cancer. Br J Radiol. 2015;88:20150197.
67. Finley DS, Belldegrun AS. Salvage cryotherapy for radiation-recurrent prostate cancer: out-comes and complications. Curr Urol Rep. 2011;12:209.
68. Bahn DK, Lee F, Silverman P, et al. Salvage cryosurgery for recurrent prostate cancer after radiation therapy: a seven-year follow-up. Clin Prostate Cancer. 2003;2:111.
69. Spiess PE, Katz AE, Chin JL, et al. A pretreatment nomogram predicting biochemical failure after salvage cryotherapy for locally recurrent prostate cancer. BJU Int. 2010;106:194.
70. Jones JS, Rewcastle JC, Donnelly BJ, et al. Whole gland primary prostate cryoablation: initial results from the cryo on-line data registry. J Urol. 2008;180:554.
71. Eisenberg ML, Shinohara K. Partial salvage cryoablation of the prostate for recurrent prostate cancer after radiotherapy failure. Urology. 2008;72:1315.
72. Spiess PE, Lee AK, Leibovici D, et al. Presalvage prostate-specific antigen (PSA) and PSA doubling time as predictors of biochemical failure of salvage cryotherapy in patients with locally recurrent prostate cancer after radiotherapy. Cancer. 2006;107:275.
73. Kanthabalan A, Peters M, Van Vulpen M, et al. Focal salvage high-intensity focused ultrasound in radiorecurrent prostate cancer. BJU Int. 2017;120(2):246–56.
74. Gelet A, Chapelon JY, Poissonnier L, et al. Local recurrence of prostate cancer after external beam radiotherapy: early experience of salvage therapy using high-intensity focused ultraso-nography. Urology. 2004;63:625.
75. Uddin Ahmed H, Cathcart P, Chalasani V, et al. Whole-gland salvage high-intensity focused ultrasound therapy for localized prostate cancer recurrence after external beam radiation ther-apy. Cancer. 2012;118:3071.
76. Ahmed HU, Cathcart P, McCartan N, et al. Focal salvage therapy for localized prostate cancer recurrence after external beam radiotherapy: a pilot study. Cancer. 2012;118:4148.
77. Shah TT, Peters M, Kanthabalan A, et al. PSA nadir as a predictive factor for biochemical disease-free survival and overall survival following whole-gland salvage HIFU following radiotherapy failure. Prostate Cancer Prostatic Dis. 2016;19:311.
78. Rouviere O, Sbihi L, Gelet A, et al. Salvage high-intensity focused ultrasound ablation for prostate cancer local recurrence after external-beam radiation therapy: prognostic value of prostate MRI. Clin Radiol. 2013;68:661.
79. Billia M, Siddiqui KM, Chan S, et al. Assessment of histopathological features of needle biopsy in recurrent prostate cancer following salvage high-intensity focused ultrasound. Can Urol Assoc J. 2016;10:416.
80. Murat F-J, Poissonnier L, Rabilloud M, et al. Mid-term results demonstrate salvage high-intensity focused ultrasound (HIFU) as an effective and acceptably morbid salvage treatment option for locally radiorecurrent prostate cancer. Eur Urol. 2009;55:640.
81. Warmuth M, Johansson T, Mad P. Systematic review of the efficacy and safety of high-intensity focussed ultrasound for the primary and salvage treatment of prostate cancer. Eur Urol. 2010;58:803.
82. Ost P, Bossi A, Decaestecker K, et al. Metastasis-directed therapy of regional and distant recur-rences after curative treatment of prostate cancer: a systematic review of the literature. Eur Urol. 2015;67:852.

83. Ost P, Jereczek-Fossa BA, As NV, et al. Progression-free survival following stereotactic body radiotherapy for oligometastatic prostate cancer treatment-naive recurrence: a multi-institutional analysis. Eur Urol. 2016;69:9.
84. Picchio M, Berardi G, Fodor A, et al. (11)C-choline PET/CT as a guide to radiation treatment planning of lymph-node relapses in prostate cancer patients. Eur J Nucl Med Mol Imaging. 2014;41:1270.
85. Casamassima F, Masi L, Menichelli C, et al. Efficacy of eradicative radiotherapy for limited nodal metastases detected with choline PET scan in prostate cancer patients. Tumori. 2011;97:49.
86. Jilg CA, Rischke HC, Reske SN, et al. Salvage lymph node dissection with adjuvant radiotherapy for nodal recurrence of prostate cancer. J Urol. 2012;188:2190.
87. Herr HW, O'Sullivan M. Quality of life of asymptomatic men with nonmetastatic prostate cancer on androgen deprivation therapy. J Urol. 2000;163:1743.

Chapter 9
Options After Chemotherapy for Patients with Metastatic, Castration-Resistant Prostate Cancer

Daniel J. Lee and Neal D. Shore

Clinical Case Scenario: 74-year-old man with asymptomatic metastatic castration-resistant prostate cancer (mCRPC), previously treated with 6 cycles of docetaxel and androgen deprivation therapy for bone metastases at initial diagnosis, who now presents for discussion of treatment options.

Prostate cancer (PCa) remains the most common non-cutaneous malignancy and third leading cause of cancer death in men, accounting for approximately 27,000 deaths in 2017 in the USA [1]. Depending upon the extent of screening and specific locales, 5–10% of newly diagnosed PCa patients in the USA present with metastatic disease, and upward of 40% of patients undergoing interventional therapy for localized disease will experience disease progression [2]. Androgen deprivation (ADT) has been the historical mainstay for advanced PCa patients [3]. Invariably, patients will eventually develop resistance to ADT and clinically progress, despite suppressing testosterone production via the endocrine axis. There are numerous mechanisms which may explain the pathophysiologic evolution to castration-resistant prostate cancer (CRPC) including amplification of the androgen receptor (AR), mutations in the AR, bypass mechanisms in the AR, or transformation to an AR-negative anaplastic variant disease which may also be associated with neuroendocrine differentiation. CRPC may ensue approximately 1–3 years after initiating ADT, and patients with CRPC have attained an average survival of about 30–34 months [4], when reviewing the most recent CRPC phase III trial publications [5–8].

D. J. Lee, M.D. (✉)
Department of Urology, Vanderbilt University Medical Center, Nashville, TN, USA
e-mail: daniel.lee.1@vanderbilt.edu

N. D. Shore, M.D., F.A.C.S.
Carolina Urologic Research Center, Myrtle Beach, SC, USA
e-mail: nshore@gsuro.com

© Springer International Publishing AG, part of Springer Nature 2018
S. S. Chang, M. S. Cookson (eds.), *Prostate Cancer*,
https://doi.org/10.1007/978-3-319-78646-9_9

The historical poor quality of life and prognosis for CRPC patients promulgated extensive research with the goal of identifying therapeutic agents capable of survival prolongation. In 2004, two seminal phase III clinical trials demonstrated a survival advantage with the use of docetaxel chemotherapy in men with metastatic CRPC (mCRPC) [9]. Until 2010, there were no therapies that were shown to have a survival benefit for patients who had post docetaxel-progressive CRPC [10]. Since 2010, five novel therapies have been approved that may confer a survival benefit for docetaxel-progressive CRPC. Sipuleucel-T is an autologous immunotherapy which demonstrated a significant survival advantage compared to placebo in asymptomatic and minimally symptomatic mCRPC patients [11] and received Federal Drug Administration (FDA) approval in April 2010. Cabazitaxel, a novel taxane that demonstrated a survival advantage over mitoxantrone [12], was FDA approved in June 2010 for men with mCRPC that progressed after docetaxel therapy. Abiraterone acetate demonstrated a survival advantage [13] and was FDA approved in April 2011 for treatment of mCRPC after docetaxel therapy. Enzalutamide was similarly found to have a survival advantage [14] and was FDA approved for treatment of docetaxel-refractory mCRPC in August 2012. Radium-223 also demonstrated a survival advantage in this setting [15] and was FDA approved for treatment of docetaxel-refractory mCRPC in May 2013.

Recent phase III trials have demonstrated improvement in overall survival for abiraterone [5, 6] and chemohormonal therapy (ADT + docetaxel) [7, 8] as first-line therapies in the treatment of metastatic hormone-sensitive prostate cancer. However, this review focuses on the contemporary management of docetaxel-progressive mCRPC, specifically when chemohormonal therapy is initiated for a newly diagnosed patient with metastatic disease in the context of guidelines that supported both FDA and European Medicines Agency approvals [16–19]. To accomplish this, an English-language literature search was performed in the electronic databases of Medline (PubMed), Embase, Web of Science, Google Scholar, and the Cochrane Library. Information regarding ongoing clinical trials was obtained from the United States National Institute of Health's website www.clinicaltrials.gov for information. The last search was performed on September 1, 2017. All trial designs were included, and all articles were English language and original articles.

Background

The prevalence of CRPC has been estimated to be about 18% among patients with prostate cancer in the USA [20]. Simulated models have predicted that the incidence of metastatic CRPC in the USA may continue to increase to about 42,970 cases in 2020, accounting for about 20% of the deaths in all men diagnosed with prostate cancer [21]. In the UK, the estimated incidence was approximately 3.8 per 100 person-years among all men diagnosed with prostate cancer [22]. About 10–20% of patients with metastatic prostate cancer eventually develop CRPC within 5 years, and about 15–30% of patients with nonmetastatic CRPC will develop metastases within 2 years [20, 22–24]. The median overall survival for asymptomatic mCRPC has also changed from 2009 to 2017, from approximately 19 months to 34 months [25, 26].

Mechanisms of Docetaxel Resistance

The success of any systemic therapy is influenced by the tumor microenvironment. Resistance to docetaxel can develop in areas of the tumor with poor blood flow and subsequent failure drug circulatory delivery that could impair effective tumoricidal drug distribution. In addition, areas of hypoxia that stimulate the production of hypoxia-inducible transcription factors can influence the expression of genes that increase treatment resistance, survivability, and metastatic potential of tumor cells [27, 28]. Docetaxel has a strong affinity for a drug efflux pump that can be overexpressed in settings of docetaxel-refractory CRPC [29]. Docetaxel triggers cell death by binding to tubulin and ultimately disrupts cell division. Docetaxel resistance can occur with alterations to the microtubule structure that prevents binding [30]. In addition, docetaxel in prostate cancer patient can induce overexpression of anti-apoptotic proteins such as Bcl-2 that will inhibit cell death and promote prostate cancer cell proliferation [31].

Treatment Options for Docetaxel-Refractory Metastatic CRPC

Given the multiple ways that resistance to ADT and docetaxel can develop among patient with prostate cancer, it is essential to have novel therapeutic options that address those mechanisms. The next sections will review emerging treatment options for metastatic CRPC.

Androgen Synthesis Inhibitors

Abiraterone Acetate

Abiraterone acetate is an oral, selective inhibitor of androgen synthesis by inhibiting17-α-hydroxylase and C17,20-lyase [32]. The phase III randomized, double-blind, placebo-controlled trial COU-AA-301 compared 1000 mg abiraterone acetate with prednisone against placebo and prednisone in men with metastatic CRPC who had previous progressed on docetaxel therapy (Table 9.1) [13]. The primary endpoint was overall survival. On the initial report with a median follow-up of 12.8 months, a significant survival advantage was seen for patients taking the

Table 9.1 Summary of approved therapeutic agents used in docetaxel-refractory castration-resistant prostate cancer

Therapeutic agent	Mechanism	Notable side effects	Dose and frequency	Route of administration	Survival benefit over placebo	Relative reduction in risk of death (%)
Abiraterone acetate	Inhibits CYP17, blocks androgen synthesis	Hepatotoxicity, hypokalemia, hypertension, gastrointestinal problems	1000 mg daily	Oral	4.6 months (15.8 vs. 11.2)	26
Enzalutamide	Inhibits androgen receptor and AR translocation	Seizures, posterior reversible encephalopathy syndrome, hypertension, fatigue, gastrointestinal problems	160 mg daily	Oral	4.8 months (18.4 vs. 13.6)	37
Cabazitaxel	Microtubule inhibitor	Hematologic abnormalities; neutropenia, thrombocytopenia, anemia, gastrointestinal problems	25 mg/m^2 every 3 weeks	Intravenous	2.4 months (15.1 vs. 12.7)	30
Radium-223	α emitting radionuclide	Bone marrow suppression, hematologic abnormalities: neutropenia, thrombocytopenia, anemia, gastrointestinal problems	55 kBq/kg body weight every 4 weeks with 6 injections	Intravenous	3.6 months (14.9 vs. 11.3)	29

abiraterone acetate (14.8 months vs. 10.9 months; hazard ratio 0.65; 95% confidence interval (CI) 0.54–0.77). On the final analysis, before unblinding and crossover at a median follow-up time of 20.2 months, a significant survival advantage was maintained for those on abiraterone acetate compared to the prednisone arm (15.8 months vs. 11.2 months; hazard ratio 0.74; 95% CI 0.64–0.86), corresponding to a survival advantage of 4.6 months and a 26% relative reduction in the risk of death [33]. In addition, abiraterone prolonged time to PSA progression (8.5 months vs. 6.6 months; $p < 0.0001$) and radiologic progression-free survival (5.6 months vs. 3.6 months; $p < 0.0001$) and had a higher proportion of patients with a PSA response (29.5% vs. 5.5%; $p < 0.0001$) compared to placebo.

In a subset analysis of symptomatic patients with metastatic docetaxel-refractory CRPC in the COU-AA-301 trial [34], abiraterone acetate was associated with improved palliation and pain control (45% vs. 28.8%, $p < 0.001$) and faster median time to palliation of pin (5.6 months vs. 13.7 months; $p = 0.002$) compared to placebo. Therefore, the AUA guidelines recommend abiraterone acetate for symptomatic metastatic CRPC with previous docetaxel therapy with good performance status [16, 17].

Overall, abiraterone acetate was well tolerated in the trials [33], with the most common grade 3–4 adverse events being fatigue (9% abiraterone vs. 10% placebo), anemia (8% vs. 8%), back pain (7% vs. 10%), and bone pain (6% vs. 8%). Mineralocorticoid-related adverse events were higher with abiraterone acetate than placebo, with higher incidence of fluid retention or peripheral edema (33% abiraterone vs. 24% placebo), hypokalemia (18% vs. 9%), hepatotoxicity (11% vs. 9%), and cardiac disorders (16% vs. 12%). Most of the mineralocorticoid-related adverse events were grade 1 or 2 adverse events, and the most frequently observed cardiac events were grade 1–2 tachycardiac events or grade 1–3 atrial fibrillation. There were higher rates of fluid retention, and hepatotoxicity with abiraterone acetate in comparison to the prednisone arm, thus prescribing abiraterone acetate in patients with liver disease, cardiac disease, or congestive heart failure, requires consideration of alternative therapies [35].

Ketoconazole

High-dose ketoconazole (800–1200 mg daily) acts as a nonselective competitive inhibitor of several cytochrome P450 enzymes including CYP-11A and CYP-17A [36]. Ketoconazole may be administered at an oral dose of 400 mg daily with hydrocortisone. Several studies have found that ketoconazole can cause ≥50% decline in PSA in about 30–60% of patients, improved radiographic response rates, and median progression-free duration of approximately 5–8 months [37–41]. Importantly, there are no phase III trials demonstrating a survival prolongation benefit from ketoconazole. The toxicities associated with ketoconazole can be difficult to manage for some patients, with about 22% of the patients experiencing a grade 3–4 toxicity [41]. The most frequent toxicities are often fatigue, anorexia, emesis, peripheral neuropathy, and transaminitis, with most patients requiring concurrent hydrocortisone. One retrospective study found that prior response to ADT, the pre-treatment PSA doubling time, and extent of disease were associated with the likeli-hood of response with ketoconazole and were factors that can be used to help evaluate the risk to benefit ratio for initiating ketoconazole. Although the response rate is lower and the incidence of toxicities is higher with ketoconazole compared to abiraterone acetate, ketoconazole is a viable alternative for patients unable to get other first-line therapies such as abiraterone acetate and is listed in the AUA guidelines [16, 17].

Androgen Receptor Blockers

Enzalutamide

Enzalutamide is an oral nonsteroidal antiandrogen that competitively inhibits andro-gen binding to the receptor, impedes nuclear translocation of the AR, prevents DNA binding, and inhibits coactivator recruitment. The AFFIRM trial was a phase III, double-blind, placebo-controlled trial that investigated the efficacy of enzalutamide compared to placebo in improving overall survival in men with metastatic CRPC after chemotherapy [14]. At a median follow-up of 14.4 months, enzalutamide was associated with increased overall survival benefit (18.4 months vs. 13.6 months; hazard ratio 0.63; 95% CI 0.53–0.75), corresponding to an overall survival benefit of 4.8 months and a 37% relative reduction in the risk of death. In addition, all sec-ondary endpoints favored enzalutamide over placebo, including the proportion of patients with $\geq$50% reduction in PSA (54% vs. 2%, $p < 0.0001$), soft-tissue response rate (29% vs. 4%, $p < 0.001$), quality of life response rate (43% vs. 18%, $p < 0.001$), time to PSA progression (8.3 months vs. 3.0 months, hazard ratio 0.40; $p < 0.001$), and time to first skeletal-related event (SRE, 16.7 months vs. 13.3 months; hazard ratio 0.69; $p < 0.001$). Subsequent analyses of the AFFIRM data showed that enzalu-tamide conferred significant advantages over placebo in improving the overall qual-ity life and decreasing pain severity [42, 43]. Patients on enzalutamide had longer median times to first SRE (16.7 months vs. 13.3 months; HR 0.69; 95% CI 0.57–0.84), lower rates of pain progression (28% vs. 39%, $p = 0.0018$), more pain pallia-tion (45% vs. 7%, $p = 0.0079$), and overall improvement in health-related quality of life (42% vs. 15%, $p < 0.0001$).

In addition, enzalutamide was well tolerated, with a relatively acceptable side effect profile. In the AFFIRM trial [14], the enzalutamide group had a lower inci-dence of grade 3 or worse adverse events compared to placebo (45.3% vs. 53.1%). Of the adverse events that were more common with enzalutamide, the most com-mon toxicities reported were fatigue (34% enzalutamide vs. 29% placebo), diarrhea (21% vs. 18%), hot flashes (20% vs. 10%), musculoskeletal pain (14% vs. 10%), headaches (12% vs. 6%), and hypertension (6.6% vs. 3.3%). There was no differ-ence in cardiac disorders (6% enzalutamide vs. 8% placebo) or hepatotoxicity. Of note, five patients (0.6%) that received enzalutamide had seizures compared to no patients in the placebo arm. No differences were noted in the incidence of seizures in the subsequent PREVAIL study [44]. Although enzalutamide is well tolerated, caution should be used when using enzalutamide in patients with a history of seizures, stroke, or uncontrolled blood pressure issues. Enzalutamide is recommended for use in patients with asymptomatic or symptomatic metastatic CRPC after chemotherapy and with good performance status [16, 17]. Enzalutamide can also be used in men with poor performance status; however, most of the men in the AFFIRM trial had good performance status.

Chemotherapy

Cabazitaxel

Cabazitaxel is a novel semisynthetic taxane that binds tubulin but differs from docetaxel and paclitaxel in its poor affinity for P-glycoprotein, the drug efflux pump [45]. The TROPIC trial was a phase III, open-label, randomized trial comparing cabazitaxel to mitoxantrone in men with metastatic CRPC who had previously received docetaxel [12]. At a median follow-up of 12.8 months, cabazitaxel use was associated with an increased overall survival benefit compared to mitoxantrone (15.1 months vs. 12.7 months; hazard ratio 0.70; 95% CI 0.59–0.83), corresponding to an increased overall survival of 2.4 months and a 30% relative reduction in the risk of death. In the TROPIC trial, the survival benefit of cabazitaxel persisted even if the men had measurable disease or pain at baseline or whether progression of disease occurred during docetaxel therapy or during a drug holiday. In subset analyses, the survival benefit was higher for those with better performance status (ECOG 0–1 vs. 2), older patients (≥65 years vs. <65 years), rising PSA at study entry, received at least 12 cycles of docetaxel previously, and for patients with disease progression within 3 months of docetaxel initiation. These findings indicate that cabazitaxel is effective even if patients have rapid disease progression early during docetaxel therapy. The side effect profile for cabazitaxel was similar to docetaxel, including significant grade 3 or worse neutropenia (82%) and leukopenia (68%) for those on cabazitaxel. Other common toxicities were diarrhea (47%), fatigue (37%), nausea (34%), and vomiting (23%). Of note, 14% of patients undergoing cabazitaxel developed peripheral neuropathy, but only 1% had grade 3 or worse neuropathy. Due to the efficacy of cabazitaxel in the docetaxel-refractory metastatic CRPC setting, the AUA guidelines recommend cabazitaxel with co-administration with neutrophil growth factor support [16, 17].

Docetaxel Re-treatment

Before the emergence of cabazitaxel and other agents in 2010 for the treatment of docetaxel-refractory metastatic CRPC, reintroduction of docetaxel after a chemotherapy holiday has been proposed as an alternative treatment strategy. Evidence from phase II trials suggests that select groups of patients who develop progression after docetaxel may benefit from a rechallenge with docetaxel. This approach was found to be beneficial especially among patients who had an initial favorable response on docetaxel, with PSA, radiographic or pain improvement, who stopped docetaxel therapy because of toxicity or after completing 10 treatment cycles [46–48]. In phase II trials with CRPC patients that had previous responses with docetaxel lasting ≥4 months, a rechallenge with docetaxel produced ≥50% declines in PSA in 25–45% of patients and radiographic improvement in about 10% and conferred a median overall survival of approximately 13–15 months and progression-free survival of 5–6 months [47, 48]. In addition, patients with a long interval (3 months or more) between the last docetaxel cycle and subsequent progression were found to have a better response with docetaxel re-treatment compared to those with a shorter interval (progression-free survival 6.3 months vs. 3.4 months; $p = 0.04$) [49].

Radionuclide Therapy

Radium-223

Radium-223 is a targeted alpha emitter and a bone-seeking calcium mimetic, which will preferentially bind to areas of high bone turnover, such as sites of bone metastases, and emit high-energy alpha particles of a shallower range given the large kilodalton alpha particle size in comparison to beta and gamma particles, thereby liming marrow penetration and the risk of myelosuppressive effects [15]. The targeted alpha therapy (TAT) Ra-223 is administered intravenously every 4 weeks for a total of six cycles. The ALSYMPCA trial was a phase III, randomized, double-blind trial comparing radium-223 against placebo in men with bone metastases and CRPC [15]. Of note, 57% of the cohort received previous docetaxel. Radium-223 was associated with a significant overall survival advantage (median 14.9 months vs. 11.3 months; hazard ratio 0.70; 95% CI 0.58–0.83), corresponding to a survival advantage of 3.6 months and a 30% relative risk reduction in death.

In a subset analysis of patients who received previous docetaxel therapy, the overall survival advantage was maintained (hazard ratio 0.71; 95% CI 0.56–0.89), corresponding to a 29% relative risk reduction with radium-223 usage group [50]. Patients who had received previous docetaxel and had radium-223 showed a significant risk reduction in the time to first SRE (median 5.8 months vs. 3.7; hazard ratio 0.62; 95% CI 0.46–0.82) and significant increase in time to PSA progression (median 3.5 months vs. 3.3 months; hazard ratio 0.74; 95% CI 0.59–0.93).

Overall, radium-223 was well tolerated, with those who had previous docetaxel and radium-223 experiencing a higher incidence of grade 3–4 thrombocytopenia (9%) compared to placebo (3%) [50]. Other common adverse events included anemia (35%), diarrhea (25%), nausea (40%), vomiting (24%), and fatigue (27%). Due to the efficacy of radium-223 and low toxicity profile, the AUA guidelines recommend radium-223 use in patients with CRPC and bone metastases, no known visceral metastasis, and good performance status, regardless of docetaxel use [50].

Treatment to Decrease Skeletal-Related Events

Men with metastatic CRPC are at risk for bone complications because of their advanced age and long-term exposure to ADT. In prospective studies of men on ADT, bone mineral density declined approximately 3% in the lumbar spine and 2% at the hip in the first year of ADT [51–54]. Furthermore, close to 90% of men with metastatic CRPC will have radiographically detectable bony metastases [9, 55]. Bony fractures can have a significant impact on the individual's quality of life and life span. For example, in elderly patients with hip fractures, 50% will have permanent functional disability, 15–25% will require long-term nursing home care, and up to 20% will die within the year [56–58]. Preventing skeletal morbidity has become an area of much investigation because of the potential impact on survival and quality of life for men with metastatic CRPC.

Vitamin D and Calcium

Multiple randomized controlled trials evaluating the association between vitamin D intake and fracture risk revealed conflicting data and information. A meta-analysis was performed to over 9000 patients, 60 years of age or older, from 7 randomized controlled trials of oral vitamin D supplementation [59]. The meta-analysis found that higher doses of vitamin D (700–800 IU/day) decreased the relative risk of hip fractures by 26%, but no significant benefit for lower doses (400 IU/day).

Hypocalcemia is a potential side effect from zoledronic acid and denosumab therapy, and calcium supplements are often given along with those therapies and vitamin D. However, calcium supplementation alone (500–1000 mg/day) has not been shown to prevent bone mineral density loss from ADT use [60]. In addition, intake of calcium may be associated with severe consequences, as some studies have found an increased risk of myocardial infarction, stroke [61, 62], and prostate cancer mortality [63]. Therefore, it is important that providers understand these risks and benefits before making recommendations for their use.

Bisphosphonates

Bisphosphonates were the first and most commonly prescribed group of osteoclast-targeting agents. The structure of bisphosphonates is similar to pyrophosphate, a normal component of bone, so that when they are incorporated into the bone matrix they prevent osteoclast-mediated bone resorption and directly inhibit osteoblasts [64]. Several bisphosphonates have been found to improve bone mineral density in men receiving ADT including zoledronic acid [53, 65], neridronate [66], pamidronate [54, 67], and alendronate [52]. However, zoledronic acid is the only bisphosphonate that showed a benefit in patients with metastatic CRPC [68]. In a placebo-controlled, randomized clinical trial, zoledronic acid reduced the risk of SRE by 36% (risk ratio 0.64; 95% CI 0.485–0.845) and was associated with a longer time to the first SRE (488 days vs. 321 days; $p = 0.009$). Although not statistically significant, there was a trend toward improved overall survival with zoledronic acid compared to placebo (546 days vs. 464 days; $p = 0.091$). Overall the zoledronic acid was well tolerated, with low incidences of hypocalcemia, nephrotoxicity, and osteonecrosis of the jaw. Due to the toxicity profile, it has been recommended that serum creatinine and calcium be obtained prior to each dose so that appropriate dose modifications and supplements can be administered [68]. Although osteonecrosis of the jaw occurs infrequently, it is associated with significant morbidity. Risk factors for developing osteonecrosis of the jaw include dental extractions during therapy, intensity of dosing, and duration of therapy [69]. An advisory task force from the American Association of Oral and Maxillofacial Surgeons recommended risk reduction by having an oral examination before starting therapy, extracting teeth before initiating therapy, and waiting about 2–3 weeks after extracting teeth before initiating therapy [70].

RANK Ligand

RANK ligand plays a central role in the regulation of osteoclast activity. Denosumab is a monoclonal antibody against RANK ligand and inhibits osteoclast-mediated bone destruction. In a randomized placebo-controlled study of patients with non-metastatic hormone-sensitive prostate cancer undergoing ADT [71], denosumab was associated with increased bone mineral density in the lumbar spine (5.6% gain vs. 1.0% loss; $p < 0.001$), hip, femoral neck, and distal radius. In addition, there was a 62% risk reduction of new vertebral fractures at 36 months (relative risk 0.38; 95% CI 0.19–0.78).

With such a potent response, a subsequent randomized trial compared denosumab to zoledronic acid in over 1900 with metastatic CRPC [72]. The trial showed that denosumab was associated with a longer time to first SRE compared to zoledronic acid (20.7 months vs. 17.1 months; hazard ratio 0.82; 95% CI 0.71–0.95). Overall survival and disease progression were equivalent between denosumab and zoledronic acid. Men treated with denosumab had significantly higher incidence of hypocalcemia (12.8% vs. 5.8%) and a nonsignificant trend toward higher osteonecrosis of the jaw (2.3% vs. 1.3%; $p = 0.09$). Because of the toxicity profile, it is important to monitor hypocalcemia before initiating denosumab and during treatment and follow similar precautions to avoid osteonecrosis of the jaw as with zoledronic acid [70].

Conclusions

The management of metastatic CRPC continues to rapidly evolve. Over the past decade, multiple large trials have provided level I evidence for an improvement in overall survival among men with docetaxel-refractory CRPC with four different agents: cabazitaxel, abiraterone acetate, enzalutamide, and radium-223. In addition, the use of vitamin D, denosumab, and zoledronic acid have been found to improve bone health and decrease the morbidity associated with skeletal fractures associated with treatment. Future research to discover and enhance optimization of sequencing and combination strategies as well as new therapeutic modalities should continue to improve the quality of life and prolong survival for men with metastatic CRPC.

References

1. Siegel RL, Miller KD, Jemal A. Cancer statistics, 2017. CA Cancer J Clin. 2017;67:7–30.
2. Shariat S, Kattan M, Vickers A, Karakiewicz P, Scardino P. Critical review of prostate cancer predictive tools. Future Oncol. 2009;5:1555–84.
3. Harzstark A, Small E. Castrate-resistant prostate cancer: therapeutic strategies. Expert Opin Pharmacother. 2010;11:937–45.
4. Lassi K, Dawson N. Emerging therapies in castrate-resistant prostate cancer. Curr Opin Oncol. 2009;21:260–5.
5. James ND, de Bono JS, Spears MR, et al. Abiraterone for prostate cancer not previously treated with hormone therapy. N Engl J Med. 2017;377:338–51.
6. Fizazi K, Tran N, Fein L, et al. Abiraterone plus prednisone in metastatic, castration-sensitive prostate cancer. N Engl J Med. 2017;377:352–60.
7. Sweeney CJ, Chen YH, Carducci M, et al. Chemohormonal therapy in metastatic hormone-sensitive prostate cancer. N Engl J Med. 2015;373:737–46.
8. James ND, Sydes MR, Clarke NW, et al. Addition of docetaxel, zoledronic acid, or both to first-line long-term hormone therapy in prostate cancer (STAMPEDE): survival results from an adaptive, multiarm, multistage, platform randomised controlled trial. Lancet. 2016;387:1163–77.
9. Petrylak DP, Tangen CM, Hussain MH, et al. Docetaxel and estramustine compared with mitoxantrone and prednisone for advanced refractory prostate cancer. N Engl J Med. 2004;351:1513–20.
10. Tannock IF, Osoba D, Stockler MR, et al. Chemotherapy with mitoxantrone plus prednisone or prednisone alone for symptomatic hormone-resistant prostate cancer: a Canadian randomized trial with palliative end points. J Clin Oncol. 1996;14:1756–64.
11. Kantoff PW, Higano CS, Shore ND, et al. Sipuleucel-T immunotherapy for castration-resistant prostate cancer. N Engl J Med. 2010;363:411–22.
12. de Bono JS, Oudard S, Ozguroglu M, et al. Prednisone plus cabazitaxel or mitoxantrone for metastatic castration-resistant prostate cancer progressing after docetaxel treatment: a randomised open-label trial. Lancet. 2010;376:1147–54.
13. de Bono JS, Logothetis CJ, Molina A, et al. Abiraterone and increased survival in metastatic prostate cancer. N Engl J Med. 2011;364:1995–2005.
14. Scher HI, Fizazi K, Saad F, et al. Increased survival with enzalutamide in prostate cancer after chemotherapy. N Engl J Med. 2012;367:1187–97.
15. Parker C, Nilsson S, Heinrich D, et al. Alpha emitter radium-223 and survival in metastatic prostate cancer. N Engl J Med. 2013;369:213–23.

16. Cookson MS, Roth BJ, Dahm P, et al. Castration-resistant prostate cancer: AUA Guideline. J Urol. 2013;190:429–38.
17. Cookson MS, Lowrance WT, Murad MH, Kibel AS, Association AU. Castration-resistant prostate cancer: AUA guideline amendment. J Urol. 2015;193:491–9.
18. Heidenreich A, Bastian PJ, Bellmunt J, et al. EAU guidelines on prostate cancer. Part II: treatment of advanced, relapsing, and castration-resistant prostate cancer. Eur Urol. 2014;65:467–79.
19. Mohler JL, Armstrong AJ, Bahnson RR, et al. Prostate cancer, version 1.2016. J Natl Compr Cancer Netw. 2016;14:19–30.
20. Alemayehu B, Buysman E, Parry D, Becker L, Nathan F. Economic burden and healthcare utilization associated with castration-resistant prostate cancer in a commercial and Medicare advantage US patient population. J Med Econ. 2010;13:351–61.
21. Scher HI, Solo K, Valant J, Todd MB, Mehra M. Prevalence of prostate cancer clinical states and mortality in the United States: estimates using a dynamic progression model. PLoS One. 2015;10:e0139440.
22. Hirst CJ, Cabrera C, Kirby M. Epidemiology of castration resistant prostate cancer: a longitudinal analysis using a UK primary care database. Cancer Epidemiol. 2012;36:e349–53.
23. Kirby M, Hirst C, Crawford ED. Characterising the castration-resistant prostate cancer population: a systematic review. Int J Clin Pract. 2011;65:1180–92.
24. Smith MR, Kabbinavar F, Saad F, et al. Natural history of rising serum prostate-specific antigen in men with castrate nonmetastatic prostate cancer. J Clin Oncol. 2005;23:2918–25.
25. Patrikidou A, Loriot Y, Eymard JC, et al. Who dies from prostate cancer? Prostate Cancer Prostatic Dis. 2014;17:348–52.
26. Omlin A, Pezaro C, Mukherji D, et al. Improved survival in a cohort of trial participants with metastatic castration-resistant prostate cancer demonstrates the need for updated prognostic nomograms. Eur Urol. 2013;64:300–6.
27. Semenza GL. Defining the role of hypoxia-inducible factor 1 in cancer biology and therapeutics. Oncogene. 2010;29:625–34.
28. Maxwell PJ, Gallagher R, Seaton A, et al. HIF-1 and NF-kappaB-mediated upregulation of CXCR1 and CXCR2 expression promotes cell survival in hypoxic prostate cancer cells. Oncogene. 2007;26:7333–45.
29. Borst P, Evers R, Kool M, Wijnholds J. A family of drug transporters: the multidrug resistance-associated proteins. J Natl Cancer Inst. 2000;92:1295–302.
30. Verrills NM, Po'uha ST, Liu ML, et al. Alterations in gamma-actin and tubulin-targeted drug resistance in childhood leukemia. J Natl Cancer Inst. 2006;98:1363–74.
31. Yamanaka K, Rocchi P, Miyake H, et al. Induction of apoptosis and enhancement of chemosensitivity in human prostate cancer LNCaP cells using bispecific antisense oligonucleotide targeting Bcl-2 and Bcl-xL genes. BJU Int. 2006;97:1300–8.
32. O'Donnell A, Judson I, Dowsett M, et al. Hormonal impact of the 17alpha-hydroxylase/C(17,20)-lyase inhibitor abiraterone acetate (CB7630) in patients with prostate cancer. Br J Cancer. 2004;90:2317–25.
33. Fizazi K, Scher HI, Molina A, et al. Abiraterone acetate for treatment of metastatic castration-resistant prostate cancer: final overall survival analysis of the COU-AA-301 randomised, double-blind, placebo-controlled phase 3 study. Lancet Oncol. 2012;13:983–92.
34. Logothetis CJ, Basch E, Molina A, et al. Effect of abiraterone acetate and prednisone compared with placebo and prednisone on pain control and skeletal-related events in patients with metastatic castration-resistant prostate cancer: exploratory analysis of data from the COU-AA-301 randomised trial. Lancet Oncol. 2012;13:1210–7.
35. Hoy SM. Abiraterone acetate: a review of its use in patients with metastatic castration-resistant prostate cancer. Drugs. 2013;73:2077–91.
36. Trachtenberg J, Zadra J. Steroid synthesis inhibition by ketoconazole: sites of action. Clin Invest Med. 1988;11:1–5.
37. Small EJ, Baron AD, Fippin L, Apodaca D. Ketoconazole retains activity in advanced prostate cancer patients with progression despite flutamide withdrawal. J Urol. 1997;157:1204–7.

38. Small EJ, Baron A, Bok R. Simultaneous antiandrogen withdrawal and treatment with ketoconazole and hydrocortisone in patients with advanced prostate carcinoma. Cancer. 1997;80(9):1755.
39. Harris KA, Weinberg V, Bok RA, Kakefuda M, Small EJ. Low dose ketoconazole with replacement doses of hydrocortisone in patients with progressive androgen independent prostate cancer. J Urol. 2002;168:542–5.
40. Johnson DE, Babaian RJ, von Eschenbach AC, Wishnow KI, Tenney D. Ketoconazole therapy for hormonally refractive metastatic prostate cancer. Urology. 1988;31:132–4.
41. Keizman D, Huang P, Carducci MA, Eisenberger MA. Contemporary experience with ketoconazole in patients with metastatic castration-resistant prostate cancer: clinical factors associated with PSA response and disease progression. Prostate. 2012;72:461–7.
42. Fizazi K, Scher HI, Miller K, et al. Effect of enzalutamide on time to first skeletal-related event, pain, and quality of life in men with castration-resistant prostate cancer: results from the randomised, phase 3 AFFIRM trial. Lancet Oncol. 2014;15:1147–56.
43. Cella D, Ivanescu C, Holmstrom S, Bui CN, Spalding J, Fizazi K. Impact of enzalutamide on quality of life in men with metastatic castration-resistant prostate cancer after chemotherapy: additional analyses from the AFFIRM randomized clinical trial. Ann Oncol. 2015;26:179–85.
44. Beer TM, Armstrong AJ, Rathkopf DE, et al. Enzalutamide in metastatic prostate cancer before chemotherapy. N Engl J Med. 2014;371:424–33.
45. Galsky MD, Dritselis A, Kirkpatrick P, Oh WK. Cabazitaxel. Nat Rev Drug Discov. 2010;9:677–8.
46. Eymard JC, Oudard S, Gravis G, et al. Docetaxel reintroduction in patients with metastatic castration-resistant docetaxel-sensitive prostate cancer: a retrospective multicentre study. BJU Int. 2010;106:974–8.
47. Beer TM, Ryan CW, Venner PM, et al. Intermittent chemotherapy in patients with metastatic androgen-independent prostate cancer: results from ASCENT, a double-blinded, randomized comparison of high-dose calcitriol plus docetaxel with placebo plus docetaxel. Cancer. 2008;112:326–30.
48. Di Lorenzo G, Buonerba C, Faiella A, et al. Phase II study of docetaxel re-treatment in docetaxel-pretreated castration-resistant prostate cancer. BJU Int. 2011;107:234–9.
49. Loriot Y, Massard C, Gross-Goupil M, et al. The interval from the last cycle of docetaxel-based chemotherapy to progression is associated with the efficacy of subsequent docetaxel in patients with prostate cancer. Eur J Cancer. 2010;46:1770–2.
50. Hoskin P, Sartor O, O'Sullivan JM, et al. Efficacy and safety of radium-223 dichloride in patients with castration-resistant prostate cancer and symptomatic bone metastases, with or without previous docetaxel use: a prespecified subgroup analysis from the randomised, double-blind, phase 3 ALSYMPCA trial. Lancet Oncol. 2014;15:1397–406.
51. Saylor PJ, Lee RJ, Smith MR. Emerging therapies to prevent skeletal morbidity in men with prostate cancer. J Clin Oncol. 2011;29:3705–14.
52. Greenspan SL, Nelson JB, Trump DL, Resnick NM. Effect of once-weekly oral alendronate on bone loss in men receiving androgen deprivation therapy for prostate cancer: a randomized trial. Ann Intern Med. 2007;146:416–24.
53. Michaelson MD, Kaufman DS, Lee H, et al. Randomized controlled trial of annual zoledronic acid to prevent gonadotropin-releasing hormone agonist-induced bone loss in men with prostate cancer. J Clin Oncol. 2007;25:1038–42.
54. Smith MR, McGovern FJ, Zietman AL, et al. Pamidronate to prevent bone loss during androgen-deprivation therapy for prostate cancer. N Engl J Med. 2001;345:948–55.
55. Tannock IF, de Wit R, Berry WR, et al. Docetaxel plus prednisone or mitoxantrone plus prednisone for advanced prostate cancer. N Engl J Med. 2004;351:1502–12.
56. Chrischilles EA, Butler CD, Davis CS, Wallace RB. A model of lifetime osteoporosis impact. Arch Intern Med. 1991;151:2026–32.
57. Magaziner J, Hawkes W, Hebel JR, et al. Recovery from hip fracture in eight areas of function. J Gerontol A Biol Sci Med Sci. 2000;55:M498–507.
58. Cummings SR, Kelsey JL, Nevitt MC, O'Dowd KJ. Epidemiology of osteoporosis and osteoporotic fractures. Epidemiol Rev. 1985;7:178–208.

59. Bischoff-Ferrari HA, Willett WC, Wong JB, Giovannucci E, Dietrich T, Dawson-Hughes B. Fracture prevention with vitamin D supplementation: a meta-analysis of randomized controlled trials. JAMA. 2005;293:2257–64.
60. Datta M, Schwartz GG. Calcium and vitamin D supplementation during androgen deprivation therapy for prostate cancer: a critical review. Oncologist. 2012;17(9):1171.
61. Lind L, Skarfors E, Berglund L, Lithell H, Ljunghall S. Serum calcium: a new, independent, prospective risk factor for myocardial infarction in middle-aged men followed for 18 years. J Clin Epidemiol. 1997;50:967–73.
62. Li K, Kaaks R, Linseisen J, Rohrmann S. Associations of dietary calcium intake and calcium supplementation with myocardial infarction and stroke risk and overall cardiovascular mortality in the Heidelberg cohort of the European Prospective Investigation into Cancer and Nutrition study (EPIC-Heidelberg). Heart. 2012;98:920–5.
63. Schwartz GG, Skinner HG. A prospective study of total and ionized serum calcium and time to fatal prostate cancer. Cancer Epidemiol Biomark Prev. 2012;21:1768–73.
64. Rogers MJ, Watts DJ, Russell RG. Overview of bisphosphonates. Cancer. 1997;80:1652–60.
65. Smith MR, Eastham J, Gleason DM, Shasha D, Tchekmedyian S, Zinner N. Randomized controlled trial of zoledronic acid to prevent bone loss in men receiving androgen deprivation therapy for nonmetastatic prostate cancer. J Urol. 2003;169:2008–12.
66. Morabito N, Gaudio A, Lasco A, et al. Neridronate prevents bone loss in patients receiving androgen deprivation therapy for prostate cancer. J Bone Miner Res. 2004;19:1766–70.
67. Diamond TH, Winters J, Smith A, et al. The antiosteoporotic efficacy of intravenous pamidronate in men with prostate carcinoma receiving combined androgen blockade: a double blind, randomized, placebo-controlled crossover study. Cancer. 2001;92:1444–50.
68. Saad F, Gleason DM, Murray R, et al. Long-term efficacy of zoledronic acid for the prevention of skeletal complications in patients with metastatic hormone-refractory prostate cancer. J Natl Cancer Inst. 2004;96:879–82.
69. Hoff AO, Toth BB, Altundag K, et al. Frequency and risk factors associated with osteonecrosis of the jaw in cancer patients treated with intravenous bisphosphonates. J Bone Miner Res. 2008;23:826–36.
70. Advisory Task Force on Bisphosphonate-Related Ostenonecrosis of the Jaws, American Association of Oral and Maxillofacial Surgeons. American Association of Oral and Maxillofacial Surgeons position paper on bisphosphonate-related osteonecrosis of the jaws. J Oral Maxillofac Surg. 2007;65:369–76.
71. Smith MR, Egerdie B, Hernández Toriz N, et al. Denosumab in men receiving androgen-deprivation therapy for prostate cancer. N Engl J Med. 2009;361:745–55.
72. Fizazi K, Carducci M, Smith M, et al. Denosumab versus zoledronic acid for treatment of bone metastases in men with castration-resistant prostate cancer: a randomised, double-blind study. Lancet. 2011;377:813–22.

Chapter 10
Evaluation and Treatment for High-Risk Prostate Cancer

Lucas W. Dean and Karim A. Touijer

Clinical Case Scenario: 58-year-old, PSA 32, Gleason 4 + 4 = 8, cT3, with single enlarged pelvic lymph node but no other evidence of metastatic disease who desires aggressive therapy.

In this case discussion, we will consider an otherwise healthy 58-year-old man with high-risk prostate cancer, serum PSA of 32 ng/mL, and clinical evidence of regional lymph node metastasis. A digital rectal exam reveals a bulky prostate with bilateral nodularity, but does not appear to be fixed in the pelvis. A standard 12-core transrectal ultrasound (TRUS)-guided systematic biopsy is performed, demonstrating 10 of 12 cores involved by Gleason 4 + 4 = 8 prostate cancer. Seventy-five percent of biopsy tissue is involved by cancer. A multiparametric MRI is performed, and a Prostate Imaging Reporting and Data System (PIRADSv2) score of 5 is assigned, with multifocal prostate tumor and bilateral extracapsular extension. A staging contrast-enhanced pelvic CT scan demonstrates a single enlarged 1.2-cm lymph node in the left obturator fossa. A bone scan is performed and is unremarkable. The patient desires aggressive therapy and recounts that his father underwent a radical prostatectomy at the age of 67.

L. W. Dean, M.D. · K. A. Touijer, M.D. (✉)
Urology Service, Department of Surgery, Memorial Sloan Kettering Cancer Center, Sidney Kimmel Center for Prostate and Urologic Cancers, New York, NY, USA
e-mail: deanl@mskcc.org; touijerk@mskcc.org

© Springer International Publishing AG, part of Springer Nature 2018   135
S. S. Chang, M. S. Cookson (eds.), *Prostate Cancer*,
https://doi.org/10.1007/978-3-319-78646-9_10

Evaluation

Risk Stratification and Prognosis

The American Joint Committee on Cancer (AJCC) TNM staging system and the National Comprehensive Cancer Network (NCCN) Risk Groups provide standardized nomenclature for prostate cancer risk stratification [1, 2]. By these criteria, our case patient has cT3 N1M0 disease, categorizing him as metastatic due to the enlarged pelvic lymph node on imaging. Approximately 12% of patients are categorized as N1 at the time of diagnosis [3]. A wealth of evidence exists for predicting prostate cancer-specific mortality (PCSM) in clinically localized disease, with multiple nomograms available for use in this setting [4, 5]. Certainly, with clinically node-positive disease, prognosis is adversely affected, though prognostic data is limited due to the relative rarity of this disease presentation. Muralidhar and colleagues recently reported on 5-year conditional survival in men with stage IV prostate cancer [6]. At diagnosis, men with N1 disease had a 5-year PCSM rate of 18.9%. After 5 years of survival, the chance of dying from prostate cancer over the subsequent 5 years was 21%. Conditional survival predictions provide important information to patients as they move through the survivorship process. Importantly, patients with N1 disease did not experience any reduction in PCSM until beyond 10 years.

Staging Evaluation

The long-held standard imaging modality to detect prostate cancer nodal metastasis is contrast-enhanced CT scan. Staging imaging is generally indicated in men with cT3 or T4 tumors or in those with a nomogram-predicted probability of lymph node involvement >10% [2]. Recently, pelvic MRI has been demonstrated to be equivalent to CT in this regard. When compared to staging lymphadenectomy, the gold standard in identifying lymph node metastasis, the performance characteristics of either of these cross-sectional imaging modalities are underwhelming. In a systematic review including 24 studies, the pooled sensitivity and specificity of CT were 42% and 82%, respectively. The reported pooled sensitivity and specificity of MRI were 39% and 82% [7]. The majority of metastatic lymph nodes involved by prostate cancer are smaller than 8 mm, contributing to these low detection rates on morphological imaging [8].

Technetium-99 (Tc-99) radionuclide bone scan is the standard for detecting bony metastases in prostate cancer. Staging evaluation with bone scan is indicated in men with an increased risk of occult metastasis (T1 and PSA >20 ng/mL, T2 and PSA >10 ng/mL, Gleason ≥8, T3–T4, or symptomatic) [2]. Interest in alternative imaging strategies to detect bony disease, including F18-sodium fluoride (NaF) PET and axial skeleton or whole-body MRI, has grown recently. NaF has a higher affinity for bone than conventional Tc-99m-methylene diphosphonate, thus allowing earlier imaging acquisition and improved image quality [9]. One study compared four different bone imaging modalities (NaF PET, NaF PET/CT, Tc-99 planar scintigraphy, single-photon emission CT [SPECT]), each performed on the same day in 44 men with high-risk prostate cancer [10]. NaF PET/CT outperformed all other modalities, with both sensitivity and specificity of 100%; however significant false-positive rates have been reported in other series [11, 12].

The diagnostic performance of contemporary MRI in detecting bone metastasis was evaluated in a recent systematic review [13]. Regardless of the coverage of the MRI—pelvis-only in routine prostate MRI, axial skeleton, or whole-body MRI— the per-patient sensitivity and specificity were consistently high (pooled sensitivity 96%, pooled specificity 98%). While these alternative imaging strategies have demonstrated promising results, they have not become standard practice, partly due to concerns regarding cost and accessibility.

Numerous molecular imaging studies, including choline-C11, fluciclovine-F18, and prostate-specific membrane antigen (PSMA)-PET, have become available in recent years. ^{68}Ga-HBED-iPSMA has quickly become the front-runner as a PSMA imaging technology in prostate cancer, given its rapid clearance and excellent signal-to-noise ratio. The main clinical applications of this—and many other molecular imaging agents thus far—have been in localizing recurrent prostate cancer after definitive local therapy and in guiding subsequent salvage radiotherapy or salvage node dissection. Interest has also been generated in using ^{68}Ga-PSMA-PET in the initial staging evaluation for prostate cancer. One retrospective study evaluated this imaging modality in 130 men with intermediate- and high-risk prostate cancer who underwent radical prostatectomy and pelvic lymph node dissection (PLND) [14]. Sensitivity of 65.9% and specificity of 98.9% were reported. Patients with pathologically positive lymph nodes but a negative PSMA-PET either harbored PSMA-negative tumors or had micrometastases in single lymph nodes. Additional protocols are underway to further evaluate the performance characteristics of PSMA-PET as a primary staging modality (NCT02611882, NCT02919111). Other molecular imaging agents are under study, including radiogallium-labeled gastrin-releasing peptide receptor prior to radical prostatectomy, in a phase II trial underway at Memorial Sloan Kettering Cancer Center (MSKCC) (NCT02559115).

Our case patient appears to have clinically node-positive disease (cN1) based on staging CT scan. The addition of further molecular imaging is not currently considered a standard of care in this setting. In the near future, molecular imaging may have a role in helping to direct therapy, be it via real-time intraoperative alterations to template-based lymphadenectomy during radical prostatectomy, or by defining targets for radiation therapy, or coupled with a treatment agent as a theranostic.

Prostate MRI

Over the last decade, uses of multiparametric MRI (mpMRI) have been developed for multiple clinical applications in prostate cancer. While it has predominantly found use in lesion characterization and targeted biopsy, mpMRI has also been enthusiastically adopted by many urologists for surgical planning prior to prostatectomy. Conceptually, this "road map" of the prostate and tumor(s) may afford improved oncologic control by allowing surgeons to modify their technique. This theory was tested in a randomized trial among 438 men who underwent a preoperative MRI prior to radical prostatectomy [15]. MRI did not reduce the overall risk of positive surgical margins, though this trial has been criticized for its use of a 1.5-Tesla magnet without an endorectal coil, potentially resulting in inferior image quality.

Multiparametric MRI does appear to be the best available tool to predict extraprostatic extension (EPE) at radical prostatectomy. When Somford and coworkers performed 3-Tesla mpMRI with an endorectal coil on 183 men prior to radical prostatectomy, the overall staging accuracy in predicting EPE was 73.8% [16], making it superior to any other preoperative parameters. The negative predictive value for EPE was very high (87.7%) for low-risk disease but dropped to 57.1% in the intermediate-risk cohort. This high false-negative rate may render mpMRI less useful in planning for nerve sparing in the intermediate-risk population. A second study showed that mpMRI altered decision-making regarding nerve sparing in approximately one-quarter of patients [17]. Synthesizing the available evidence, a recent Cancer Care Ontario clinical practice guideline concluded that mpMRI for pretreatment local staging exhibited only modest imaging performance [18]. The authors qualified any recommendation due to design limitations and variability in reported outcomes among the studies analyzed.

Genetic Testing

Recently published data show that men with metastatic prostate cancer may have germline mutations in one of 16 DNA repair genes at a rate of 11.8% [19]. While node-positive patients were not specifically analyzed, the rate of germline DNA repair mutations in men with localized high-risk prostate cancer was 6%. Additional data show that DNA repair mutations may occur at a high rate in metastatic castration-resistant prostate cancer [20] and that patients with these germline mutations may have an improved response to PARP inhibition therapy [21]. The NCCN Guidelines panel recommends inquiring about personal and family history of cancer and considering germline testing for those with high- or very high-risk clinically localized or metastatic prostate cancer [2]. While genetic testing is not currently considered a standard of care, it would be reasonable to pursue in our case patient since the genomic data in prostate cancer is developing rapidly.

Therapeutic Management

Overview

The historical attitude toward node-positive prostate cancer, whether clinically positive on preoperative imaging (cN+) or pathologically on biopsy or staging lymphadenectomy (pN+), was to avoid local therapy. This long-held concept has recently been challenged. In the contemporary setting, regional lymph node involvement does not preclude definitive local therapy. Node-positive disease does not always equate to systemic disease; thus a proportion of N1M0 patients have potentially curable disease, in distinction to those with M1 prostate cancer. This is an important distinction given that N1M0 and M1 patients are collectively lumped together as stage IV. In selected N1 cases, radical prostatectomy or radiotherapy may be considered to treat the primary tumor and lymph nodes.

Abdollah and colleagues analyzed data from the National Cancer Database on the usage of local therapy in men with clinical lymph node involvement [22]. They found that either radical prostatectomy or radiation therapy was performed two-thirds of the time. Five-year overall survival favored men who received local therapy plus ADT vs. ADT alone (78.8% vs. 49.2%). Instrumental variable analysis did not show a difference in survival between those men who underwent radical prostatectomy compared to radiation therapy. Mounting retrospective data support the delivery of definitive local therapy with high-risk and/or node-positive prostate cancer. Though not the focus of this chapter, several prospective protocols are underway to investigate the role of definitive local therapy in men with oligometastatic disease. Despite enthusiasm for this aggressive approach, it cannot be considered a standard of care at this time and should be carefully individualized.

Androgen Deprivation Therapy Alone

Historically, men with node-positive prostate cancer were often placed solely on ADT, the rationale being that these men had disseminated disease and would not benefit from local therapy. The European Organisation for Research and Treatment of Cancer (EORTC) 30846 trial provides insight into the role of ADT alone in node-positive prostate cancer [23]. A total of 234 men with histologically confirmed lymph node metastasis (N1-3; 1972 TNM classification) were randomized to immediate ADT versus delayed ADT initiated upon clinical disease progression. These patients had originally been diagnosed with localized prostate cancer and scheduled for radical prostatectomy, but prostatectomy was abandoned when node-positive disease was identified at pelvic lymphadenectomy. Final results at a median follow-up of 13 years, reported in 2009, showed the 10-year PCSM was not significantly different: 52.1% in the immediate ADT group vs. 55.6% in the delayed ADT group. These results demonstrated that, in men with node-positive prostate cancer, immediate ADT alone without local therapy was not superior to ADT initiated upon clinical progression. From this study and other contemporary data that showed benefits to local therapy, it can be seen that the predicted outcomes of treating node-positive disease with ADT alone are poor [21, 23–25]. As further argument for definitive local therapy in this patient population, the newer systemic therapies targeting the androgen receptor axis have failed to demonstrate durable long-term survival when applied in node-positive and metastatic prostate cancer [26].

Radical Prostatectomy

Surgical Considerations

Historically, a staging lymphadenectomy was often performed prior to radical prostatectomy, at which time the operation was aborted if frozen sections identified nodal metastasis. This practice has been abandoned, based largely on the German experience showing that men treated with ADT fared poorly compared to men who had the prostatectomy completed [23]. In contemporary urologic practice, radical prostatectomy is increasingly performed for high- and very high-risk clinically localized prostate cancer, often as the initial component of what will likely be multimodal therapy [27]. In general, a PLND is performed in virtually all men with intermediate or higher-risk disease [2]. There remains significant debate over the anatomic boundaries of the procedure and whether or not there is any therapeutic benefit of removing involved nodes. The performance of an extended PLND may identify positive lymph nodes when the nodes within a limited template are negative [28]. Unfortunately, the only randomized trial supporting the use of extended PLND was retracted due to data falsification [29]. Of men with lymph node metastasis identified at the time of PLND, approximately one-third remain free of disease at 10 years without any additional treatment [30]. Despite this observational evidence, there are no randomized data to show that PLND improves survival. Given our case patient's single positive node on preoperative imaging, there is a significant likelihood that other lymph nodes harbor microscopic foci of cancer. An extended lymph node dissection should be carried out. The dissection is typically bounded by the external iliac vein anteriorly, pelvic side wall laterally, bladder wall medially, floor of the pelvis posteriorly, Cooper's ligament distally, and internal iliac artery proximally. As discussed in the prior section on *Staging Evaluation*, molecular imaging may be used in the future to direct the lymphadenectomy, to include anatomic regions not typically dissected. Until then, we rely on template-based approaches.

Results

Several retrospective series have been published on men with node-positive prostate cancer treated with radical prostatectomy. One of the largest comes from the Munich Cancer Registry, in which Engel and colleagues reviewed the outcomes of 688 men with positive nodes who underwent prostatectomy and lymphadenectomy and compared them to 250 men in whom the radical prostatectomy was abandoned once the positive nodes were identified [24]. The 10-year overall survival for patients who underwent prostatectomy was 63.8%, compared to 28.2% for men who did not undergo prostatectomy (p-value not reported) (Table 10.1). Two other retrospective studies of similar methodology, in which men underwent a bilateral PLND with frozen sections, have been reported. Men who went on to receive a radical prostatectomy had better prostate cancer-specific survival than those who did not [31, 32]. However, these nonrandomized analyses [24, 31, 32] are limited by the likely potential that younger and healthier men were more likely to have had a radical prostatectomy completed.

A proportion of men with pathologic lymph node involvement discovered at the time of radical prostatectomy will remain free of disease without post-prostatectomy therapy. Touijer and colleagues retrospectively reviewed 369 men with lymph node metastasis discovered at the time of radical prostatectomy and pelvic lymphadenectomy. They found that approximately a third remained free of disease at 10 years without any additional treatment [30]. The predicted 10-year overall and cancer-specific survival rates were 60% and 72%, respectively. Furthermore, those with only one or two positive nodes represented a favorable group that enjoyed improved disease-free survival relative to those with more extensive nodal involvement.

While not directly applicable to our case patient with nodal-only disease, there are several ongoing prospective trials evaluating the use of radical prostatectomy in combination with systemic therapy in men with oligometastatic prostate cancer (NCT02716974, NCT02742675, NCT01751438). These trials should provide high-quality evidence informing the role of surgical local therapy and may question the long-held notion that metastatic prostate cancer should only be treated with systemic therapy.

Neoadjuvant Therapy Prior to Radical Prostatectomy

Zurita and colleagues from MD Anderson Cancer Center reported phase II data on the feasibility of neoadjuvant ADT and docetaxel followed by consolidative RP [33]. This study included men presenting with clinically detected lymph node metastases or with features in the primary tumor portending a very high risk for lymph node involvement. ADT was combined with three cycles of docetaxel chemother-

Table 10.1 Comparative studies reporting outcomes of radical prostatectomy in node-positive prostate cancer

Authors	Design	No. of subjects	Median follow-up (years)	Overall survival	Cancer-specific survival	Recurrence-free survival	Notes
Radical prostatectomy vs. conservative management							
Steuber (2011) [31]	Retrospective, single center	158	8.2	NR	(10-year) RP completed: 76% RP aborted: 46% (p = 0.001)	(10-year) RP completed: 61% RP aborted: 31% (p = 0.005)	Compared outcomes of men who had RP completed vs. those whose RP was aborted after staging LND
Engel (2010) [24]	Retrospective, Munich Cancer Registry	938	5.6	(10-year) RP completed: 64% RP aborted: 28% (p-value NR)	(10-year relative survival) RP completed: 86% RP aborted: 40% (p-value NR)	NR	Compared outcomes of men who had RP completed vs. those whose RP was aborted after staging LND
Frohmuller (1995) [32]	Retrospective, single center	139	4.5	(10-year) RP completed: 51% RP aborted: 30% (p = 0.07)	(10-year) RP completed: 71% RP aborted: 32% (p = 0.002)	(10-year) RP completed: 36% RP aborted: 15% (p = 0.002)	Compared outcomes of men who had RP completed vs. those whose RP was aborted after staging LND

Adjuvant ADT vs. observation

		N	Follow-up			(PFS)	
Messing (2006) [34]	Randomized trial, multicenter (ECOG 3886)	98	11.9	Adjuvant ADT: median 13.9 years	Adjuvant ADT: not reached		Randomized men with pN+ after RP to immediate ADT vs. delayed ADT initiated on clinical progression
				Observation: median 11.3 years	Observation: median 12.3 years	Favored adjuvant ADT	
				(p = 0.04)	(p = 0.0001)	(HR 3.42, p < 0.0001)	

Adjuvant RT vs. no RT

		N	Follow-up				
Kaplan (2013) [38]	Retrospective, SEER-Medicare data	577	NR	RT: 5.1 deaths/100 patient-years	RT: 2.9 deaths/100 patient-years	NR	Propensity score models used to compare outcomes for men who did and did not receive adjuvant RT within 1 year of RP
				No RT: 3.8 deaths/100 patient-years	No RT: 1.3 deaths/100 patient-years		
				(p = 0.153)	(p = 0.09)		
Briganti (2011) [64]	Retrospective, two centers	364	7.9	(10-year)	(10-year)	NR	Compared matched patients who received adjuvant RT after RP vs. those who did not
				RT: 74%	RT: 86%		
				No RT: 55%	No RT: 70%		
				(p < 0.001)	(p = 0.004)		

ADT androgen deprivation therapy, *ECOG* Eastern Cooperative Oncology Group, *HR* hazard ratio, *LND* lymph node dissection, *NR* not reported, *PFS* progression-free survival, *pN+* pathologically node-positive, *RP* radical prostatectomy, *RT* radiotherapy, *SEER* surveillance, epidemiology and end results apy. Patients with a PSA <1 ng/mL at the end of the 1-year systemic treatment period were then offered radical prostatectomy with extended PLND. Over half the patients had cN1 disease at enrollment, with another 18% having clinical evidence of nonregional lymph node involvement (M1a). Out of 39 evaluable patients, 26 (67%) underwent surgery. Half of those who underwent surgery were progression free at 1 year postoperatively. Treatment failure was defined as objective tumor progression, PSA ≥1 ng/mL, or any postoperative radiation, hormonal, or other systemic therapy. At a median follow-up of 61 months, median time to treatment failure was 27 months in these men who had undergone surgery. Four men had a PSA that remained undetectable at last follow-up. Despite lacking a comparative arm of men who received ADT only, this study demonstrated the feasibility of consolidative surgery in selected men with a good response to neoadjuvant systemic therapy.

Adjuvant Androgen Deprivation Therapy After Radical Prostatectomy

In a well-known landmark study, Messing et al. randomized patients with pathologically positive nodes at the time of radical prostatectomy and PLND to immediate ADT versus ADT instituted at the time of disease progression (Table 10.1) [34]. Ninety-eight men were randomized between 1988 and 1993. The long-term results were published in 2006, at a median follow-up of 11.9 years. Patients in the immediate ADT arm had a longer median overall survival than men in the delayed ADT arm (13.9 years vs. 11.3 years, $p = 0.04$). While this trial provides level 1 evidence to support the use of immediate ADT in men with pathological node involvement at the time of radical prostatectomy, it has come under some criticism. Two commonly cited problems include the trial's small size and the fact that men in the delayed ADT arm died at a higher rate than would be expected based on other contemporaneous series of node-positive men [35]. Clinical trials are underway using newer androgen receptor axis therapies as adjuvant therapy after radical prostatectomy in those with high-risk pathology, including lymph node involvement (NCT01927627).

Adjuvant Radiotherapy After Radical Prostatectomy

Multiple retrospective series have investigated the role of adjuvant radiotherapy (RT) in addition to ADT in men with lymph node invasion at radical prostatectomy. The most compelling data was published by Abdollah and colleagues in 2014 [36]. Men with pN1 prostate cancer who underwent radical prostatectomy and extended PLND between 1988 and 2010 were analyzed ($n = 1107$). On multivariate analysis, the 35% of men who underwent adjuvant RT had a more favorable PCSM rate (HR 0.37, $p < 0.001$). When stratified into risk groups, men with ≤2 positive nodes and another adverse pathologic feature (Gleason score 7–10, pT3b/T4 stage, or positive margin) and patients with 3–4 positive nodes benefitted from the addition of adjuvant RT. A collaborative effort between MSKCC, Mayo Clinic, and the San Raffaele Hospital in Milan investigated the optimal adjuvant treatment strategy for men with node-positive prostate cancer after radical prostatectomy [37]. Management strategies included observation, ADT alone, or ADT plus external beam radiation therapy (EBRT) and were chosen by provider and institutional preference. Cancer-specific and overall survival benefits were demonstrated for men who underwent adjuvant ADT + EBRT, despite these patients having the highest proportion of pT4 disease, Gleason grade 8–10, and positive surgical margins. These results supporting adjuvant RT are contradicted by Kaplan and coworkers, however, who published a propensity-adjusted analysis based on SEER data (Table 10.1) [38]. Men who underwent adjuvant RT within 1 year of prostatectomy ($n = 177$) were compared to those who did not ($n = 400$). Adjuvant RT was not associated with differences in overall or cancer-specific survival. Given this contradictory evidence on adjuvant RT after prostatectomy in those with lymph node involvement, further randomized trials are needed.

It is interesting to examine how patients with node-positive prostate cancer are most commonly managed after radical prostatectomy in a contemporary setting. Zareba and colleagues utilized the National Cancer Database to describe patterns of care and outcomes of nearly 8000 men found to have lymph node metastasis at the time of radical prostatectomy [39]. The majority of men (63%) were initially managed with observation alone, while 20% were managed with ADT, 5% with RT, and 13% with both ADT and RT. Use of multimodality therapy increased over time, with 15% of men receiving combined ADT + RT in 2014, compared to 8% in 2004. Those with adverse pathology, including higher stage tumors and positive surgical margins, were also more likely to receive combination therapy. On multivariate analysis, the combination of ADT + RT was associated with lower all-cause mortality compared to observation alone (HR 0.69, 95% CI 0.52–0.92, $p = 0.010$) and ADT alone (HR 0.65, 95% CI 0.48–0.89, $p = 0.008$). Treatment with either ADT or RT alone resulted in overall survival similar to that of the observation group. These findings echo the results of other observational data, supporting a benefit to multimodality therapy in this high-risk group.

Definitive Radiotherapy

Treatment Considerations

Radiotherapy techniques have evolved over recent decades to deliver higher doses of radiation in a safe manner. Intensity-modulated radiation therapy (IMRT) has become a standard, allowing the radiation dose to conform more closely to the three-dimensional shape of the target. For conventionally fractionated external beam radiotherapy (EBRT), total doses up to 81.0 Gy are typically administered to the prostate [40]. Moderately hypofractionated IMRT regimens (in which higher doses per fraction are delivered over a shorter duration) are increasingly being used and have been evaluated in four randomized trials [41–44]. Overall, with medium-term follow-up, there appears to be similar efficacy to conventional fractionation without an increase in toxicity. Stereotactic body RT (SBRT) is essentially an extremely hypofractionated form of RT, in which all the treatments are administered over 5 or fewer fractions. A pooled analysis of 1100 patients from prospective phase II trials showed encouraging results for PSA relapse-free survival, though few high-risk patients were included [45].

The majority of men with high-risk or even very high-risk prostate cancer have clinically negative lymph nodes. While a standard of care has not been established, men whose nomograms predict a high-risk of lymph node involvement often receive whole-pelvis RT, though two randomized studies failed to document benefits in either progression-free survival or overall survival [46, 47]. Radiotherapy delivered to men with clinical evidence of lymph node involvement should include whole-pelvis RT. Further randomized data are needed that incorporate modern radiotherapy techniques such as hypofractionated RT and SBRT in this population.

The NCCN guidelines recommend EBRT and 2–3 years of ADT as a treatment option for N1 prostate cancer [2]. While there is level 1 evidence to support this treatment strategy in high-risk clinically localized disease [48], there are no randomized data to guide decision-making regarding RT in those with clinically node-positive disease. Multiple retrospective series provide lower-level evidence of a benefit with EBRT as local therapy in addition to ADT in node-positive patients.

Results

Zagars and colleagues published early data in 2001 on 255 men with pelvic node-positive prostate cancer treated with RT + ADT or ADT alone (Table 10.2) [49]. These men had subclinical pelvic nodal metastasis that was detected by staging pelvic lymphadenectomy. The addition of RT as a definitive local therapy was at the discretion of the urologist. The RT + ADT group had improved 10-year overall survival compared to the ADT alone group (67% vs. 46%, $p = 0.008$). The addition of prostatic RT to systemic ADT also resulted in improved local control and freedom from metastasis. SEER data have also been analyzed to try to answer the question whether definitive treatment with RT confers a benefit over ADT alone. Tward and coworkers performed a regression analysis on 1100 men with cN1 prostate cancer diagnosed between 1988 and 2006. They found that the 10-year cancer-specific survival for those who received RT was 62.7% compared to 50.3% for those who did not have local therapy. The number needed to treat to prevent one prostate cancer-specific death at 10 years was eight patients [50].

An initial publication from the control arm of the STAMPEDE trial in 2014 shed some light on the potential benefit of RT in N1M0 patients [51]. While this trial is best known for supporting the use of up-front docetaxel in the metastatic hormone-sensitive setting, it also provides nonrandomized data supporting radiotherapy in N1M0 patients. The standard-of-care control arm consisted of men with high-risk clinically localized, node-positive, or metastatic prostate cancer in whom ADT for >2 years was planned. A comparison was drawn between the node-positive patients

Table 10.2 Comparative studies reporting outcomes of radiation therapy in node-positive prostate cancer

Authors	Design	No. of subjects	Median follow-up (years)	Overall survival	Cancer-specific survival	Recurrence-free survival	Notes
RT vs. No RT							
Lin (2015) [65]	Retrospective, NCDB	636	2.7	(5-year) RT: 72% No RT: 53% ($p < 0.001$)	NR	NR	Used National Cancer Database and propensity score matching to compare the addition of EBRT to ADT alone in cN+ disease
Rusthoven (2014) [66]	Retrospective, SEER data	2991	6.8	(10-year; cN+ cohort) RT: 45% No RT: 29% ($p < 0.001$)	(10-year; cN+ cohort) RT: 67% No RT: 53% ($p < 0.001$)	NR	Used SEER data to compare EBRT to no local therapy. Two cohorts (cN+ and pN+) were analyzed separately
Tward (2013) [50]	Retrospective, SEER data	1100	7.5	(5-year) RT: 68% No RT: 56% ($p < 0.01$)	(5-year) RT: 78% No RT: 71% ($p < 0.01$)	NR	Used SEER data to compare EBRT to no local therapy in men with cN+ prostate cancer
Zagars (2011) [49]	Retrospective, single center	255	9.4	(10-year) RT: 67% No RT: 46% ($p = 0.008$)	NR	(10-year) RT: 80% No RT: 25% ($p < 0.001$)	Compared outcomes of men treated with EBRT + ADT vs. ADT alone after positive nodes identified on staging LND

(continued)

Table 10.2 (continued)

Authors	Design	No. of subjects	Median follow-up (years)	Overall survival	Cancer-specific survival	Recurrence-free survival	Notes
RT + ADT vs. RT alone							
Granfors (2006) [67]	Randomized trial	91	9.7	RT + ADT: 24% RT: 13% ($p = 0.03$)	RT + ADT: 64% RT: 43% ($p = 0.02$)	NR	Randomized men with positive lymph nodes on staging LND to RT + orchiectomy vs. RT alone
Lawton (2005) [53]	Subgroup analysis of randomized trial (RTOG 85–31)	173	6.5	(5-year) RT + ADT: 72% RT: 62% ($p = 0.03$)	NR	(5-year) RT + ADT: 54% RT: 10% ($p < 0.001$)	Subgroup analysis of biopsy-proven node-positive men randomized to RT + ADT vs. RT alone. 24% had undergone a prior RP

ADT androgen deprivation therapy, *cN+* clinically node-positive, *EBRT* external beam radiotherapy, *LND* lymph node dissection, *NCDB* National Cancer Database, *NR* not reported, *PFS* progression-free survival, *pN+* pathologically node-positive, *RP* radical prostatectomy, *RT* radiotherapy, *RTOG* Radiation Therapy Oncology Group, *SEER* surveillance, epidemiology and end results who received RT versus those who did not, showing 2-year failure-free survival rates of 85% and 55%, respectively (p-value not reported).

Several randomized trials support the addition of RT in men with locally advanced prostate cancer managed with ADT. One such trial, NCIC CTG PR.3/ MRC UK PR07, randomized 1205 men (T3/T4 prostate cancer, or organ-confined disease with either PSA >40 ng/mL or PSA >20 ng/mL and Gleason score $\geq$ 8) to RT + ADT or ADT alone [48]. The addition of RT to ADT improved overall survival at 7 years (74% vs. 66%, p = 0.033). Notably, over 80% of patients had either radiological or surgical staging of their lymph nodes, and those subjects with known lymph node involvement had been excluded from randomization. A second randomized phase III trial, SPCG-7/SFUO-3, utilized similar methodology and demonstrated a 50% reduction in 10-year PCSM [52]. Again, men with PSA $\geq$11 ng/mL had staging lymph node dissection performed, and those with nodal disease were not eligible for the trial.

Adjuvant ADT After Radiotherapy

The RTOG 85–31 trial, initiated in 1985, trialed the addition of ADT to EBRT in men with locally advanced prostate cancer. A subgroup analysis of men with histologically confirmed lymph node positivity was subsequently published, analyzing the 173 men with biopsy-proven nodal disease (Table 10.2) [53]. Ninety-eight patients received RT plus immediate ADT, and 75 received RT alone (plus ADT upon relapse). The 9-year progression-free survival was 10% for those who received immediate ADT, compared to 4% for those who received ADT only at the time of relapse (p < 0.0001). These retrospective data in node-positive men align with the available level 1 evidence, which shows a benefit of ADT in addition to RT in men with intermediate and high-risk clinically localized disease.

Chemotherapy

Multiple recently published trials have evaluated the use of docetaxel chemotherapy in castration-sensitive metastatic prostate cancer [54–56]. The STAMPEDE and CHAARTED trials demonstrated a benefit for docetaxel in this setting (Table 10.3) [51, 52]. STAMPEDE also included men with high-risk localized disease and node-positive disease [55]. Radiotherapy was optional for patients with N+M0 disease. While 14% of men randomized were N+M0 at diagnosis, the outcomes of this subgroup of patients were unfortunately not reported separately with respect to response to docetaxel. GETUG-12 randomized 413 men with high-risk localized or node-positive prostate cancer to docetaxel, estramustine, and ADT or ADT alone [57]. All patients underwent a staging pelvic lymph node dissection and subsequently underwent local therapy with radical prostatectomy or RT after initiating systemic therapy. Overall, the chemotherapy plus ADT arm had improved 8-year relapse-free

Table 10.3 Comparative studies reporting outcomes of systemic therapy in node-positive prostate cancer

Authors	Design	No. of subjects	Median follow-up (years)	Overall survival	Cancer-specific survival	Recurrence-free survival	Notes
Immediate ADT vs. Delayed ADT							
Schröder (2009) [23]	Randomized trial (EORTC 30846)	234	13	Immediate ADT: 7.6 years Delayed ADT: 6.1 years (p = NS)	(10-year) Immediate ADT: 48% delayed ADT: 44% (p = NS)	NR	Randomized men with positive lymph nodes on biopsy or LND to immediate ADT vs. delayed ADT at investigatory discretion
Chemotherapy							
James (2016) [55]	Subgroup of randomized trial (STAMPEDE)	2962	3.6	(All patients) Favored ADT + docetaxel vs. ADT alone (HR = 0.78, p = 0.006)	NR	NR	14% of men randomized were N+M0. RT as local treatment was optional for these patients. This subgroup was not reported on separately
Fizazi (2015) [57]	Randomized trial (GETUG-12)	413	8.8	NR	NR	(8-year, all patients) ADT + chemotherapy: 62% ADT alone: 50% (p = 0.017) N+ subgroup (p = NS)	Randomized men with high-risk or node-positive disease to docetaxel+estramustine+ADT vs. ADT alone. 29% were N+, sensitivity analysis crossed line-of-no-effect for this group

ADT androgen deprivation therapy, *HR* hazard ratio, *LND* lymph node dissection, *N+* node-positive, *NR* not reported, *NS* not significant, *RT* radiotherapy survival when compared to the ADT alone arm (62% vs. 50%, $p = 0.017$). While 29% of men were node-positive, the sensitivity analysis for this group of patients crossed the line-of-no-effect. Based on the reported data from these two randomized trials [55, 57], we cannot draw any reliable inferences regarding the usage of chemotherapy in the node-positive patient.

Considerations for Local Control of Symptoms

A proportion of men with advanced or untreated prostate cancer will develop significant obstructive symptoms, urinary retention, or hematuria due to untreated local tumor growth. These men may require transurethral resection for relief of outlet obstruction or treatment of prostate-related bleeding. Ureteric obstruction is also not uncommon, requiring chronic upper tract drainage with indwelling stents or percutaneous nephrostomy tubes. An older Swedish study investigated the need for these additional treatments in men with prostate cancer treated with non-curative intent [58]. They found that among men who presented with non-metastatic disease, 59% required a transurethral resection and 22% required an upper urinary tract drainage procedure over a median survival duration of 94 months. With new drug therapies prolonging survival in advanced prostate cancer in recent years, there exists an increased potential for local symptoms to develop.

Our case patient is young, with a locally advanced cT3 primary tumor and a high volume of disease on biopsy. He likely has a significant chance of requiring intervention for local symptomatic progression if treated systemically only. Wiegand and colleagues reported on 192 patients with lymph node-positive prostate cancer who underwent treatment with either radical prostatectomy, radical prostatectomy + ADT, or ADT alone [59]. Men who were treated with ADT alone had significantly higher odds of symptomatic local progression on logistic regression analysis compared to men treated with radical prostatectomy alone (OR = 8.67, $p < 0.001$). If our case patient has significant pretreatment lower urinary tract symptoms, consideration might lean toward radical prostatectomy, as data show that men with larger glands and higher International Prostate Symptom Scores (IPSS) will experience higher rates of urinary toxicity when treated with RT [60, 61].

Conclusion

The optimal management of our case patient is not based on randomized evidence, rather on clinical judgment and mounting observational evidence that definite local therapy is beneficial. While lymph node involvement at the time of diagnosis is relatively rare, it is possible that the size of this group may grow with recent decreased utilization of PSA screening. Given our case patient's young age, excellent performance status, and motivation for aggressive therapy, it is certainly reasonable to pursue local therapy. With respect to surgery versus radiotherapy, there are no randomized data to help us choose one over the other. Zelefsky et al. retrospectively evaluated the MSKCC experience and compared the effect of radical prostatectomy and EBRT on distant metastasis rates in patients with localized prostate cancer [62]. For the very high-risk subgroup, the 8-year probability of metastasis was 13% for radical prostatectomy and 30% for RT. Cooperberg et al. conducted a similar analysis using the CaPSURE registry [63]. After balancing patients through the use of the Cancer of the Prostate Risk Assessment (CAPRA) score, those with very high-risk disease had a 10-year PCSM rate of 36% for radical prostatectomy and 47% for RT. While these reports did not include those with clinical lymph node involvement, the biologic behavior of these very high-risk cancers can likely be extrapolated to this disease state. So long as our case patient's disease is not so locally advanced that it substantially involves the bladder neck or invades the pelvic floor musculature or ureters, he may be a suitable candidate for initial surgery.

Decision-making must take place in a shared fashion with the patient and ideally in a multidisciplinary setting. It is of paramount importance that patients with very high-risk clinically localized or node-positive prostate cancer understand the likelihood that they will require multimodality treatment. While node-positive patients are lumped in with widely metastatic prostate cancer as stage IV, a proportion of those with nodal metastasis can be cured by aggressive therapy and in those with lower-risk node-positive disease, up to 45% of the time with surgical monotherapy [2]. While node-positive disease has historically been treated solely with ADT, local therapy may confer a benefit separate from the time-off from hormonal therapy, which would also be a consideration in this otherwise healthy younger patient. We await guidance from clinical trials in this arena, but until then we would advocate for up-front surgical therapy, likely as a part of a risk-adapted multimodal approach.

References

1. American Joint Committee on Cancer. In: Edge SB, Byrd DR, Compton CC, Fritz AG, Greene FL, Trotti A, editors. AJCC cancer staging manual. 7th ed. New York: Springer; 2010.
2. National Comprehensive Cancer Network. NCCN Clinical Practice Guidelines in Oncology. Prostate Cancer (Version 2.2017). http://www.nccn.org/professionals/physician_gls/pdf/prostate.pdf. Accessed 31 July 2017.
3. National Cancer Institute. SEER Stat Fact Sheets: Prostate Cancer. http://seer.cancer.gov/statfacts/html/prost.html. Accessed 31 July 2017.
4. Memorial Sloan Kettering Cancer Center. Pre-Radical Prostatectomy Nomogram. https://www.mskcc.org/nomograms/prostate/pre-op. Accessed 31 July 2017.
5. Cooperberg MR, Pasta DJ, Elkin EP, et al. The University of California, San Francisco Center of the Prostate Risk Assessment score: a straightforward and reliable preoperative predictor of disease recurrence after radical prostatectomy. J Urol. 2005;173:1938–42.
6. Muralidhar V, Mahal BA, Nguyen PL. Conditional cancer-specific mortality in T4, N1, or M1 prostate cancer: implications for long-term prognosis. Radiat Oncol. 2015;10:155.

7. Hovels AM, Heesakkers RA, Adang EM, et al. The diagnostic accuracy of CT and MRI in the staging of pelvic lymph nodes in patients with prostate cancer: a meta-analysis. Clin Radiol. 2008;63:387–95.
8. Fossati N, Willemse PM, Van den Broeck T, et al. The benefits and harms of different extents of lymph node dissection during radical prostatectomy for prostate cancer: a systematic review. Eur Urol. 2017;72:84–109.
9. Segall G, Delbeke D, Stabin MG, et al. SNM practice guideline for sodium 18F-fluoride PET/CT bone scans 1.0. J Nucl Med. 2010;51:1813–20.
10. Even-Sapir E, Metser U, Mishani E, et al. The detection of bone metastases inpatients with high-risk prostate cancer: 99mTc-MDP Planar bone scintigraphy, single- and multi-field-of-view SPECT,18F-fluoride PET, and 18F-fluoride PET/CT. J Nucl Med. 2006;47:287–97.
11. Simpath SC, Sampath SC, Mosci C, et al. Detection of osseous metastasis by 18F-NaF/18F-FDG PET/CT versus CT alone. Clin Nucl Med. 2015;40:e173–7.
12. Araz M, Aras G, Küçük OZ. The role of 18F–NaF PET/CT in metastatic bone disease. J Bone Oncol. 2015;4:92–7.
13. Woo S, Suh CH, Kim SY, et al. Diagnostic performance of magnetic resonance imaging for the detection of bone metastasis in prostate cancer: a systematic review and meta-analysis. Eur Urol. 2018;73(1):81–91. https://doi.org/10.1016/j.eururo.2017.03.042.
14. Maurer T, Gschwend JE, Rauscher I, et al. Diagnostic efficacy of 68gallium-PSMA-PET compared to conventional imaging in lymph node stating of 130 consecutive patients with intermediate to high-risk prostate cancer. J Urol. 2016;195:1436–43.
15. Rud E, Baco E, Klotz D, et al. Does preoperative magnetic resonance imaging reduce the rate of positive surgical margins at radical prostatectomy in a randomized clinical trial? Eur Urol. 2015;68:487–96.
16. Somford DM, Hamoen EH, Futterer JJ, et al. The predictive value of endorectal 3 Tesla multiparametric magnetic resonance imaging for extraprostatic extension in patients with low, intermediate and high risk prostate cancer. J Urol. 2013;190:1728–34.
17. Park BH, Jeon HG, Jeong BC, et al. Influence of magnetic resonance imaging in the decision to preserve or resect neurovascular bundles at robotic assisted laparoscopic radical prostatectomy. J Urol. 2014;192:82–8.
18. Salerno J, Finelli A, Morash C, et al. Multiparametric magnetic resonance imaging for pretreatment local staging of prostate cancer: a Cancer Care Ontario clinical practice guideline. Can Urol Assoc J. 2016;10:332–9.
19. Pritchard CC, Mateo J, Walsh MF, et al. Inherited DNA-repair gene mutations in men with metastatic prostate cancer. N Engl J Med. 2016;375:443–53.
20. Robinson D, Van Allen EM, Wu YM, et al. Integrative clinical genomics of advanced prostate cancer. Cell. 2015;161:1215–28.
21. Mateo J, Carreira S, Sandhu S, et al. DNA-repair defects and olaparib in metastatic prostate cancer. N Engl J Med. 2015;373:1697–708.
22. Abdollah F, Seisen T, Vetterlein M, et al. Efficacy of local treatment in patients with prostate cancer with clinically pelvic lymph node-positive disease at initial diagnosis. J Clin Oncol. 2017;35(Suppl 6S):Abstract 164.
23. Schroder FH, Kurth KH, Fossa SD, et al. Early versus delayed endocrine treatment of T2-T3 pN1-3 M0 prostate cancer without local treatment of the primary tumor: final results of the European Organisation for the Research and Treatment of Cancer protocol 30846 after 13 years of follow-up (a randomised control trial). Eur Urol. 2009;55:14–22.
24. Engel J, Bastian PJ, Baur H, et al. Survival benefits of radical prostatectomy in lymph node-positive patients with prostate cancer. Eur Urol. 2010;57:754–61.
25. Grimm MO, Kamphausen S, Hugenschmidt H, et al. Clinical outcome of patients with lymph node positive prostate cancer after radical prostatectomy versus androgen deprivation. Eur Urol. 2002;41:628–34.
26. James ND, de Bono JS, Spears MR, et al. Abiraterone for prostate cancer not previously treated with hormone therapy. N Engl J Med. 2017;377:338–51.

27. Stattin P, Sandin F, Thomsen FB, et al. Association of radical local treatment with mortality in men with very high-risk prostate cancer: a semiecologic, nationwide, population-based study. Eur Urol. 2017;72:125–34.
28. Wawroschek F, Wagner T, Hamm M. The influence of serial sections, immunohistochemistry, and extension of pelvic lymph node dissection on the lymph node status in clinically localized prostate cancer. Eur Urol. 2003;43:132–6.
29. Ji J, Yuan H, Wang L, et al. Is the impact of the extent of lymphadenectomy in radical prostatectomy related to the disease risk? A single center prospective study. J Surg Res. 2012;178:779–84.
30. Touijer KA, Mazzola CR, Sjoberg DD, et al. Long-term outcomes of patients with lymph node metastasis treated with radical prostatectomy without adjuvant androgen-deprivation therapy. Eur Urol. 2014;65:20–5.
31. Steuber T, Budaus L, Walz J, et al. Radical prostatectomy improves progression-free and cancer-specific survival in men with lymph node positive prostate cancer in the prostate-specific antigen era: a confirmatory study. BJU Int. 2011;107:1755–61.
32. Frohmuller HG, Theiss M, Manseck A, et al. Survival and quality of life of patients with stage D1 (T1-3 pN1-2 M0) prostate cancer: radical prostatectomy plus androgen deprivation versus androgen deprivation alone. Eur Urol. 1995;27:202–6.
33. Zurita AJ, Pisters LL, Wang X, et al. Integrating chemohormonal therapy and surgery in known or suspected lymph node metastatic prostate cancer. Prostate Cancer Prostatic Dis. 2015;18:276–80.
34. Messing EM, Manola J, Yao J, et al. Immediate versus deferred androgen deprivation treatment in patients with node-positive prostate cancer after radical prostatectomy and pelvic lymphad-enectomy. Lancet Oncol. 2006;7:472–9.
35. Cadeddu JA, Partin AW, Epstein JI, et al. Stage D1 (T1-3, N1-3, M0) prostate cancer: a case-controlled comparison of conservative treatment versus radical prostatectomy. Urology. 1997;50:251–5.
36. Abdollah FR, Karnes J, Suardi N, et al. Impact of adjuvant radiotherapy on survival of patients with node-positive prostate cancer. J Clin Oncol. 2014;32:3939–48.
37. Touijer KA, Karnes JR, Passoni N, et al. Survival outcomes of men with lymph node-positive prostate cancer after radical prostatectomy: a comparative analysis of different postoperative management strategies. Eur Urol. 2017. Epub ahead of print.
38. Kaplan JR, Kowalczyk KJ, Borza T, et al. Patterns of care and outcomes of radiotherapy for lymph node positivity after radical prostatectomy. BJU Int. 2013;111:1208–14.
39. Zareba P, Eastham JA, Scardino PT, Touijer K. Contemporary patterns of care and outcomes of men found to have lymph node metastases at the time of radical prostatectomy. J Urol. 2017;198:1077–84.
40. Eade TN, Hanlon AL, Horwitz EM, et al. What dose of external-beam radiation is high enough for prostate cancer? Int J Radiat Oncol Biol Phys. 2007;68:682–9.
41. Catton CN, Lukka H, Gu CS, et al. Randomized trial of a hypofractionated radiation regimen for the treatment of localized prostate cancer. J Clin Oncol. 2017;35:1884–90.
42. Lee WR, Dignam JJ, Amin MB, et al. Randomized phase III noninferiority study comparing two radiotherapy fractionation schedules in patients with low-risk prostate cancer. J Clin Oncol. 2016;34:2325–32.
43. Dearnaley D, et al. Five year outcomes of a phase III randomised trial of conventional or hypo-fractionated high dose intensity modulated radiotherapy for prostate cancer (CRUK/06/016): report from the CHHiP trial investigators group. Abstract 8LBA, European Cancer Congress 2015. Eur J Cancer. 2015;51(suppl 3):S712.
44. Incrocci L, Wortel RC, Aluwini SA, et al. Hypofractionated vs. conventionally fractionated radiation therapy for prostate cancer: 5-year oncologic outcomes of the Dutch randomized phase 3 HYPRO trial. Abstract LBA2, ASTRO 2015. Int J Radiat Oncol Biol Phys. 2015;93(3 suppl).

45. King CR, Freeman D, Kaplan I, et al. Stereotactic body radiotherapy for localized prostate cancer: pooled analysis from a multi-institutional consortium of prospective phase II trials. Radiother Oncol. 2013;109:217–21.
46. Pommier P, Chabaud S, Lagrange JL, et al. Is there a role for pelvic irradiation in localized prostate adenocarcinoma? Preliminary results of GETUG-01. J Clin Oncol. 2007;25:5366–73.
47. Lawton CA, DeSilvio M, Roach M, et al. An update of the phase III trial comparing whole pelvic to prostate only radiotherapy and neoadjuvant to adjuvant total androgen suppression: updated analysis of RTOG 94-13, with emphasis on unexpected hormone/radiation interactions. Int J Radiat Oncol Biol Phys. 2007;69:646–55.
48. Warde P, Mason M, Ding K, et al. Combined androgen deprivation therapy and radiation therapy for locally advanced prostate cancer: a randomised, phase 3 trial. Lancet. 2011;273:2104–11.
49. Zagars GK, Pollack A, von Eschenbach AC. Addition of radiation therapy to androgen ablation improves outcome for subclinically node-positive prostate cancer. Urology. 2011;58:233–9.
50. Tward JD, Kokeny KE, Shrieve DC, et al. Radiation therapy for clinically node-positive prostate adenocarcinoma is correlated with improved overall and prostate cancer-specific survival. Pract Radiat Oncol. 2013;3:234–40.
51. James ND, Spears MR, Clarke NW, et al. Impact of node status and radiotherapy on failure-free survival in patients with newly-diagnosed non-metastatic prostate cancer: data from >690 patients in the control arm of the STAMPEDE trial. Oral abstract 18. Int J Radiat Oncol Biol Phys. 2014;90(1 suppl):S13.
52. Widmark A, Klepp O, Solber A, et al. Endocrine treatment, with or without radiotherapy, in locally advanced prostate cancer (SPCG-7/SFUO-3): an open randomised phase III trial. Lancet. 2009;373:301–8.
53. Lawton CA, Winter K, Grignon D, et al. Androgen suppression plus radiation versus radiation alone for patients with stage D1/pathologic node-positive adenocarcinoma of the prostate: updated results based on national prospective randomized trial Radiation Therapy Oncology Group 85-31. J Clin Oncol. 2005;23:800–7.
54. Sweeney CJ, Chen YH, Carducci M, et al. Chemohormonal therapy in metastatic hormone-sensitive prostate cancer. N Engl J Med. 2015;373:737–46.
55. James ND, Sydes MR, Clarke NW, et al. Addition of docetaxel, zoledronic acid, or both to first-line long-term hormone therapy in prostate cancer (STAMPEDE): survival results from an adaptive, multiarm, multistage, platform randomised controlled trial. Lancet. 2016;387:1163–77.
56. Gravis G, Boher JM, Joly F, et al. Androgen deprivation therapy (ADT) plus docetaxel versus ADT alone in metastatic non castrate prostate cancer: impact of metastatic burden and long-term survival analysis of the randomized phase 3 GETUG-AFU15 trial. Eur Urol. 2016;70:256–62.
57. Fizazi K, Faivre L, Lesaunier F, et al. Androgen deprivation therapy plus docetaxel and estramustine versus androgen deprivation therapy alone for high-risk localized prostate cancer (GETUG 12): a phase 3 randomised controlled trial. Lancet Oncol. 2015;16:787–94.
58. Aus G, Hugosson J, Norlen L. Need for hospital care and palliative treatment for prostate cancer treated with noncurative intent. J Urol. 1995;154:466–9.
59. Wiegand LR, Hernandez M, Pisters LL, et al. Surgical management of lymph-node-positive prostate cancer: improves symptomatic control. BJU Int. 2010;107:1238–42.
60. Schultheiss TE, Lee WR, Hunt MA, et al. Late GI and GU complications in the treatment of prostate cancer. Int J Radiat Oncol Biol Phys. 1997;37:3–11.
61. Harsolia A, Vargas C, Yan D, et al. Predictors for chronic urinary toxicity after the treatment of prostate cancer with adaptive three-dimensional conformal radiotherapy: dose-volume analysis of a phase II dose-escalation study. Int J Radiat Oncol Biol Phys. 2007;69:1100–9.
62. Zelefsky M, Eastham J, Cronin A, et al. Metastasis after radical prostatectomy or external beam radiotherapy for patients with clinically localized prostate cancer: a comparison of clinical cohorts adjusted for case mix. J Clin Oncol. 2010;28:1508–13.

63. Cooperberg M, Vickers A, Broering J, et al. Comparative risk-adjusted mortality outcomes after primary surgery, radiotherapy, or androgen-deprivation therapy for localized prostate cancer. Cancer. 2010;116:5226–34.
64. Briganti A, Karnes RJ, Da Pozzo LF, et al. Combination of adjuvant hormonal and radiation therapy significantly prolongs survival of patients with pT2-4 pN+ prostate cancer: results of a matched analysis. Eur Urol. 2011;59:832–40.
65. Lin CC, Gray PJ, Jemal A, et al. Androgen deprivation with or without radiation therapy for clinically node-positive prostate cancer. J Natl Cancer Inst. 2015;107:djv119.
66. Rusthoven CG, Carlson JA, Waxweiler TV, et al. The impact of definitive local therapy for lymph node-positive prostate cancer: a population-based study. Int J Radiat Oncol Biol Phys. 2014;88:1064–73.
67. Granfors T, Modiq H, Damber JE, et al. Long-term followup of a randomized study of locally advanced prostate cancer treated with combined orchiectomy and external radiotherapy versus radiotherapy alone. J Urol. 2006;176:544–7.

Chapter 11
High-Intensity Focused Ultrasound (HIFU) Options for High-Risk Prostate Cancer

Bruno Nahar, Vivek Venkatramani, and Dipen J. Parekh

Clinical Case Scenario: 64-year-old man with a PSA of 5.2, T1c DRE whose MRI biopsy and sextant biopsy reveal a single focus of Gleason 8 (4 + 4) carcinoma who desires the best focal therapy.

Prostate cancer (PCa) is the second most common cancer in men in the USA [1], and approximately 11.6% of men will be diagnosed with PCa at some point during their lifetime [2]. Although the majority of these patients are diagnosed with low-risk prostate cancer, up to 30% of men will present with high-risk PCa [3]. Given the fact that high-risk PCa is an aggressive and lethal disease, radical treatment with surgery and/or radiation therapy has been the standard of care for years. While whole-gland radical treatment provides excellent cancer control, it is associated with the potential for adverse effects with significant negative impact on patient's urinary-, sexual-, and bowel-related quality of life, depending on the modality of treatment used [4, 5].

High-intensity focused ultrasound (HIFU) was approved by the FDA in 2015 for prostate tissue ablation. HIFU ablates the prostatic tissue by delivering focused ultrasound waves through an endorectal probe. The ultrasound energy produced by the HIFU device is absorbed by the prostatic tissue and converted into heat. It can reach temperatures of up to 100 °C in a few seconds and leads to tissue necrosis [6].

The experience with HIFU started in Europe in the 1990s. Since that time, more than 65,000 patients have been treated with HIFU worldwide. However, the majority

B. Nahar, M.D. (✉) · V. Venkatramani · D. J. Parekh, M.D.
Department of Urology, University of Miami Miller School of Medicine, Miami, FL, USA
e-mail: brunonahar@miami.edu; vxv218@med.miami.edu; parekhd@med.miami.edu

© Springer International Publishing AG, part of Springer Nature 2018
S. S. Chang, M. S. Cookson (eds.), *Prostate Cancer*,
https://doi.org/10.1007/978-3-319-78646-9_11

of these patients had localized disease and were treated with whole-gland ablation. Thüroff et al. [7] reported their 15-year follow-up experience with 704 patients with localized intermediate- or high-risk disease. Among those, 281 men had high-risk disease and were treated with whole-gland HIFU. The study showed acceptable rates of biochemical-free survival (82% and 68% at 5 and 10 years, respectively) and cancer-specific survival after 15 years (99%). These results are supported by other series [8]. Despite the good oncological outcomes, only half the men retained their potency after treatment, which reflects the side effects of whole-gland treatment for the prostate.

Focal therapy (FT) of the prostate is emerging as a potential alternative for the treatment of prostate cancer by reducing the morbidity associated with whole-gland treatment. It is well known that prostate cancer is a multifocal disease; however FT relies on the premise that a single focus, called the index lesion, drives tumor growth and the risk of metastasis [9]. In fact, studies have shown that the vast majority of metastatic prostate cancer has a monoclonal origin [10]. Therefore, if the index lesion can be accurately identified and targeted, FT can provide a valuable treatment alternative for those men who wish to preserve their quality of life without jeopardizing cancer control.

Among different energy sources for FT, HIFU remains one of the most effective and safest options. The largest published data on focal HIFU ablation is a French multicenter study [11] with 111 patients, who underwent hemiablation and a mean follow-up of 2 years. The infield positive biopsy rate for any cancer was 14%. Additionally, the authors reported a 95% negative follow-up biopsy for any cancer ISUP grade ≥ 2. Furthermore, the radical treatment-free survival rate was 89% at 2 years. As expected for focal ablations, the functional outcomes were remarkably good with a 12-month continence rate of 97% and a preserved erectile function in 78% of patients. The most common complications were urinary tract infection (16%), transient dysuria (15%), urinary retention (12%), and transient perineal pain (9%). Clavien-Dindo Grade III complications were seen in 13% of patients, who required prolonged catheterization or TURP. Several other authors have demonstrated similar outcomes with focal HIFU [12].

Up to now, most focal HIFU studies have included only low- to intermediate-risk PCa, owing to the fact that these men are less likely to recur systemically, and therefore local control could be curative. However, there is no reason to believe that HIFU would not provide as effective local cancer control for high-risk cancers as it does for low to intermediate risk. Therefore, in selected patients with low-volume and high-risk PCa, focal HIFU might play an important role. Most importantly, to perform focal ablation for high-risk PCa, it is imperative to precisely determine early-stage and organ-confined disease at the time of diagnosis. Nonetheless, the NCCN guidelines, as well as the AUA and EAU guidelines, do not recommend FT for patients with high-risk cancer outside of a clinical trial as of now, due to the lack of available data [13, 14].

Diagnosis and Evaluation

Diagnosis

Transrectal Ultrasound (TRUS) and TRUS Biopsy

TRUS biopsy still remains the most widely used method to diagnose prostate cancer; however TRUS alone has an accuracy of 60% with a poor negative predictive value of only 6%. TRUS also has no ability to distinguish grade or significance of lesions, and targeting hypoechoic lesions on TRUS has a low yield. As a result, TRUS is still mainly used to facilitate a template biopsy. Even newer modifications like color Doppler and elastography have not improved the detection ability of TRUS. At present, TRUS biopsy alone is generally not recommended as a tool to select candidates for focal therapy.

Template Mapping Biopsies

To improve the poor diagnostic accuracy of TRUS, some physicians use a transperineal approach to perform systematic mapping biopsies of all quadrants of the prostate. This approach was initially used as the gold standard for selecting patients for focal therapy and is still used at many centers [15]. However, it tends to diagnose many insignificant tumors and is associated with additional morbidity. Furthermore, the procedure needs to be performed under anesthesia thereby limiting its widespread application.

Multiparametric Magnetic Resonance Imaging (mpMRI) and MR Fusion Biopsy

mpMRI is the most commonly used imaging method to localize significant prostate cancer, and the use of MRI-guided fusion biopsy has changed the paradigm in the diagnosis of patients with prostate cancer. The use of mpMRI which incorporates functional sequences like diffusion-weighted imaging, as well as contrast enhancement, has been shown to help identify clinically significant cancer within the prostate [16]. Diffusion-weighted imaging (DWI) assesses the random movement of water molecules within the prostatic tissue, showing restricted diffusion in cancerous regions. This has been shown to correlate with the presence of aggressive or higher-grade cancer within the prostate. With the use of better-quality sequences and 3-Tesla machines, an endorectal coil is usually unnecessary thereby increasing patient acceptability.

There is good evidence supporting the use of mpMRI in the diagnosis of prostate cancer. The multicenter validation PROMIS study [17] found that mpMRI had a significantly better sensitivity (93% vs. 43%, $p < 0.001$) and negative predictive value (89% vs. 74%, $p < 0.001$) than TRUS alone. This study concluded that fusion biopsy was better than regular TRUS biopsy in detecting clinically significant cancer. Other reviews [18, 19] have shown that MRI fusion biopsy has a negative predictive value for significant cancer ranging from 64 to 98%, which is better than a standard TRUS biopsy.

However, mpMRI can potentially underestimate the extent of cancer by 10–20%, which should be taken into account when planning focal therapy. A recent study showed that MRI fusion biopsy can accurately predict eligibility for focal therapy in 75% of men with intermediate-risk disease when compared to the radical prostatectomy specimen [20]. Similarly, Siddiqui et al. [21], showed that MRI fusion biopsy had a 77% concordance rate with the prostatectomy specimen compared to only 53% for standard TRUS. Furthermore, the authors analyzed the utility of targeted biopsy alone vs. combined targeted biopsy and standard biopsy and showed that the combined approach led to the diagnosis of an additional 22% of prostate cancer. Although the majority was low-risk cancer, still targeted biopsies missed 17% and 5% of intermediate- and high-risk cancers, respectively.

Taken together with the high negative predictive value, there is now a growing consensus that mpMRI together with MRI fusion biopsy provide an acceptable determination of the presence of high-grade or clinically significant prostate cancer and can be used to select patients for focal therapy of the prostate in this setting [22, 23]. However, concerns regarding the potential underestimation of the extent and aggressiveness of some cancers on mpMRI need further study and have prompted treatment margins to be larger than the lesion seen on mpMRI.

A consensus panel did express the need for a study comparing the performance of mpMRI to template mapping biopsies to determine whether mpMRI alone is adequate for patient selection [24]. The PICTURE trial was recently concluded and showed that mpMRI imaging had an AUC of 0.76 when compared to template mapping biopsies in detecting clinically significant cancer in men with prior negative biopsies. However, this can be partly explained by the fact that mpMRI has false positives and this trial did not include MRI-targeted biopsies thereby reducing the accuracy of the MRI-directed pathway [25]. Based on current data, we still recommend the combined approach of targeted and standard biopsies for optimal cancer detection on patients undergoing focal HIFU.

Staging for High-Risk Prostate Cancer

For high-risk disease, guidelines recommend local and distant staging using axial imaging (computed tomography [CT] or MRI) as well as a whole-body bone scan [13]. Local staging for high-risk prostate cancer is best performed using MRI of the prostate to detect extracapsular extension or seminal vesicle involvement. However, MRI has a low sensitivity and specificity (39% and 82%, respectively) for the detection of lymph node metastases, and CT is even worse [26]. The use of newer molecular agents in positron emission tomographic (PET) imaging shows great promise in the detection of metastases. Choline-PET CT and C11-acetate have shown high sensitivity and pooled specificity in the detection of lymph node metastases, and PSMA-directed agents also appear promising [27]. Tc-99-based bone scintigraphy is a low-cost method and remains the most widely available modality to detect bone metastases. However, it has a low accuracy. Newer agents such as F-18 NaF, F-18 acetate PET-CT, and choline-based PET-CT have shown excellent results in this setting. An alternative approach with a lower sensitivity but higher specificity than PET-CTs is whole-body MRI which easily outperforms traditional bone scans. Studies on the use of FACBC and PSMA-directed agents are also being performed.

These newer modalities hold promise to enhance diagnostic precision in the staging of high-risk disease, and may be the way forward to thoroughly evaluate potential candidates prior to consideration for treatment in general, and especially allow for selection of optimal high-risk disease candidates for focal therapy.

Molecular Markers

Lately, a number of tissue-based genomic biomarkers have entered the market for determining the genomic profile of the tumor for prognosis and potentially altering treatment decisionmaking. They claim to address prostate cancer heterogeneity allowing molecular risk stratification with the ability to individualize prostate cancer treatment. However, the data at present remains weak, and there are no head-to-head comparisons between the various tests. It is possible that in the future these tests could play a role in potentially selecting focal vs. more radical treatment in this cohort of patients.

Specific Situations and Contraindications

Prostate Anatomy

The location of the tumor and size of the prostate are very important factors in planning treatment and will be discussed subsequently. Large calcifications within the prostate can prevent the transmission of ultrasound waves through the tissue potentially limiting the efficacy of HIFU. A similarly effect may be observed with significant fluid-filled cavities or cysts (>10 cm³) within the prostate. Intraprostatic stents, permanent seed implants, or implants such as an artificial urinary sphincter or penile prosthesis may also alter the local anatomy and efficacy of treatment, and caution should be exercised in these cases. A large median lobe of the prostate is generally not within the focal distance for HIFU and is not amenable to treatment; however the probability of cancer in this area is very low.

Rectal or Anal Disease

Rectal or anal fibrosis or stenosis (e.g., secondary to prior local surgery like hemor-
rhoidectomy) can make insertion of the HIFU probe difficult, or in some cases
impossible, precluding this modality of treatment. Active inflammatory bowel disease or perianal and rectal fistulae are also potential contraindications to this
procedure.

Latex Allergy

The HIFU probe needs to be covered by a latex balloon prior to insertion into the
rectum. At present, latex is the best available material and has been shown to allow
consistent transmission of the ultrasound waves. There is no replacement available
for the Ablatherm device. However, there is a non-latex ultrasound balloon available
for the Sonablate.

Baseline Functional Evaluation

A baseline assessment of the patient's lower urinary tract symptoms (LUTS) and
sexual function is essential. At the University of Miami, we use the International
Prostate Symptom Score (IPSS) to document baseline LUTS. This allows us to
determine the potential need for concurrent BPH treatment either with medication or TURP, as well as for comparison with postoperative symptoms. We document baseline erectile function using the Sexual Health Inventory for Men
(SHIM) in order to realistically counsel patients regarding postoperative outcomes and compare postoperative scores. The short-form version of the Extended
Prostate Cancer Index Composite (EPIC-26), which is also routinely used at our
practice, is a validated questionnaire used to assess health-related quality of life
across five specific PCa domains (urinary incontinence, urinary irritative/obstruc-
tive symptoms, bowel-related side effects, sexual health, and hormonal
symptoms).

Therapeutic Management

As of today, there are three commercially available HIFU devices: Ablatherm, Focal
One (both from EDAP Technomed, Lyon, France), and Sonablate (Sonocare,
Indianapolis, IN, USA). The Focal One, which uses mpMRI imaging to target the
ablation area, is pending regulatory approval by the FDA. Although the fundamen-
tals between these devices are similar and they provide precise and accurate focal
ablation, there are some differences that need to be addressed.

The Ablatherm machine consists of two separate modules: the treatment module, which includes the patient's bed with the endorectal ultrasound probe, and the planning module, used for planning and monitoring of treatment. The system has a 7.5 MHz imaging transducer and a 3 MHz ablation transducer incorporated in a single ultrasound probe, which is fully controlled by the software. The machine has several safety features integrated, including a patient movement detector and rectal wall distance monitoring, which stop the treatment if the patient moves or the rectum is too close to the ablation area. There is also a cooling system that keeps the rectum at a temperature of 14–15 °C throughout the procedure, minimizing injuries to the rectum. However, the maximum depth that can be reached by the ultrasound waves is 24 mm, which might be a limitation for anterior lesions.

The main difference between the Focal One and the Ablatherm is that it uses mpMRI images to guide the ablation, which allow the operator to perform a precise fusion focal ablation. Furthermore, the maximum depth of the ultrasound waves has been increased to 40 mm.

The Sonablate platform has no dedicated treatment bed. It comes with several probes, which have a single transducer of 4 MHz for both imaging and treatment. These probes are selected by the operator depending on the depth of the ultrasound wave required. Sonablate can reach up to 37 mm, allowing it to reach more anterior lesions. It also has many safety features, such as monitoring the amount of energy accumulated in the rectal wall and allowing the operator to stop the treatment in order to avoid damage to the rectal wall. The Sonablate also allows the operator to adjust the total acoustic power for each individual dose of HIFU, depending on the varied characteristic of the tissue. However, the procedure is more operator dependent, since the probe has to be manually placed and manipulated by the operator. There is a HIFU fusion Platform available for the Sonablate, called Sonafusion, which integrates the Sonablate planning software with mpMRI fusion biopsy platforms.

Before discussing the therapeutic management for focal HIFU, it is important to understand the terminology regarding FT. A Delphi consensus project [28] tried to standardize many definitions on focal HIFU by providing recommendations on how to report outcomes. With regard to the type of ablation, FT was defined as any ablation (with safe margins) that is less than whole gland, including quadrant, hemiablation, bilateral subtotal, and "hockey stick."

In the setting of focal therapy, particularly for high-risk patients, it is crucial to determine the precise location of the index lesion before planning the optimal type of ablation. As discussed earlier, mpMRI and MRI-US fusion biopsies results, when available, should be used to help define the treatment plan. Since local control is mandatory for high-risk prostate cancer, we recommend performing either quadrant or hemiablation, depending on the location of the lesion. Regardless of the type of ablation, it is important to avoid positive margins. A recent study [29] showed that mpMRI underestimates the size of the prostatic lesion. By comparing the size of the lesion on the mpMRI with the radical prostatectomy specimen, the authors showed that a 9 mm margin around the lesion should be achieved to provide 100% ablation of the index lesion. This study curbed the enthusiasm on minimal focal ablation, and clinicians are trending toward more extensive focal ablations to avoid positive margins.

Among all different locations, apical lesions tend to be the most challenging. First, these lesions are more likely to be missed or underestimated on mpMRI and MRI-/US-guided biopsies [30]. Second, there is always a risk of injury to the external sphincter when ablating apical lesions. Therefore, clinicians traditionally leave a safety distance (usually 4 mm) between the anatomical apex (real apex) and the ablation apex, which is the most distal limit of the ablation and where the machine usually starts treatment. However, studies have shown that the apex is the most common site of recurrence post focal ablation. The French multicenter study [11] reported that among 33 patients with positive biopsy, 17 (51%) involved the apex. Furthermore, if we consider only positive biopsies in the treated lobe, 67% were located in the apex. At our department, we use a 2 mm safety distance for apical lesions. For lesions located at the median lobe or base, a 4 mm safety distance can be used.

One major limitation of HIFU is ablation of anterior lesions. As mentioned earlier, the maximum anterior-posterior distance reached by HIFU varies from 24 to 40 mm, depending on the platform being used. Therefore, any lesion beyond these limits might be missed during the ablation, and this is particularly true for an enlarged prostate. However, there is significant variability between the anterior-posterior distance on pre-HIFU imaging and real-time HIFU imaging, which makes it very hard to predict preoperatively whether an anterior lesion would be feasible for HIFU ablation. To overcome this problem, several authors have proposed the combined use of transurethral resection of the prostate (TURP) followed by HIFU to decrease the size of the prostate and increase the penetration depth of the ultrasound waves. Additionally, this combination significantly decreased urinary catheterization time as well as rates of urinary retention, which is one of the most common complications associated with HIFU [31, 32]. However, this approach is used more frequently for whole-gland treatment. In the FT setting, where part of the gland remains untouched, we do not believe that routine TURP is mandatory. As per our protocol, we perform TURP combined with focal HIFU on patients with a prostate gland ≥ 40 cm^3 and moderate to severe IPSS.

Follow-Up

Patients with high-risk PCa are at increased risk for local and systemic recurrence; therefore close monitoring and follow-up are necessary. We perform a mpMRI at 1 month on all patients to assess adequacy of the ablation (Fig. 11.1). Our follow-up

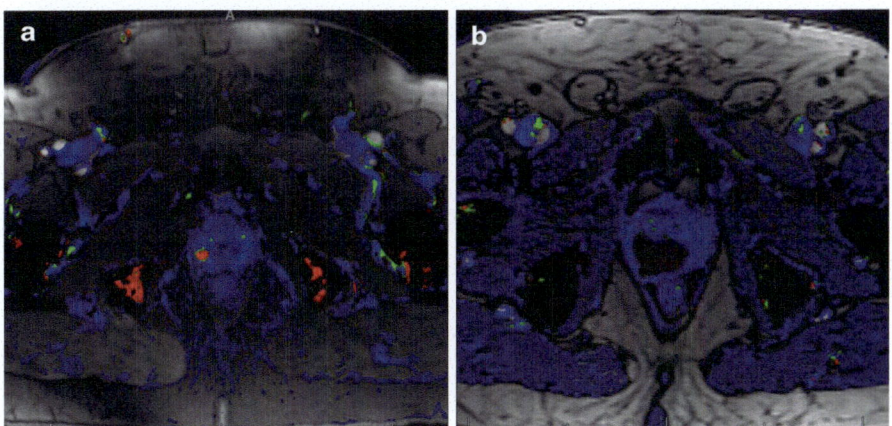

Fig. 11.1 A 76-year-old patient with a PSA of 4.2 ng/mL and Gleason 5 + 5 = 10 prostate cancer, involving two targeted biopsy cores. All other cores negative for cancer. He underwent a right quadrant HIFU ablation. 3-month PSA dropped to 0.5 ng/mL. The 6-month follow up biopsy was negative for cancer (**a**) DCE sequence showing lesion with focal contrast enhancement on mpMRI prior to HIFU. (**b**) mpMRI DCE sequence demonstrating the absence of enhancement (necrotic cavity) 1 month after focal HIFU ablation

protocol for high-risk PCa also includes PSA every 3 months and a MRI-US fusion biopsy at 6 months (12 months for intermediate and low risk). With regard to functional outcomes, IPSS, SHIM, and EPIC are collected at every 3-month follow-up visit (Table 11.1). Although the PSA levels tend to drop significantly after focal HIFU (usually below 2 ng/mL), it is not a reliable marker since a significant amount of prostatic tissue is left untreated. No definition of biochemical recurrence can be recommended based on current data. Therefore, follow-up biopsies are extremely important to define treatment success or failure. According to the Delphi Consensus project on FT [28], three possible treatment failures can occur: *ablation failure*, when there is residual cancer in the treated area due to inability of the HIFU energy to destroy it; *targeting failure*, when the energy was not correctly applied to the targeted area (i.e., anterior lesions); and *selection failure,* when the selected patient was not a candidate for FT (i.e., patients with metastatic disease missed on preoperative evaluation). For patients with ablation failure, several treatment options are accepted, including repeat HIFU, whole-gland or radical treatment with radiation therapy or surgery, and active surveillance, if eligible. On the other hand, patients with either targeting or selection failure should avoid repeat HIFU due to a high risk of second failure.

Table 11.1 The University of Miami follow-up protocol

	Baseline	Postop visit	1 month	3 month	6 month	9 month	12 month	15 month	18 month	24 month
Clinical evaluation	X	X		X	X	X	X	X	X	X
SHIM	X			X	X	X	X	X	X	X
IPSS	X			X	X	X	X	X	X	X
Epic-26	X			X	X	X	X	X	X	X
PSA	X			X	X	X	X	X	X	X
mpMRI	X		X		(X) for high risk		X			X
Confirmatory biopsy					(X) for high risk		X			

Conclusion

Radical treatment of the entire prostate gland is still the standard of care for high-risk PCa. However, focal HIFU ablation is a safe procedure and has shown promising short-term oncological outcomes, with acceptable complication rate and excellent functional outcomes. Prospective studies with long-term follow-up are needed to determine the true role of focal HIFU for PCa. Until then, focal HIFU should be offered only in the setting of clinical trials, particularly for high-risk PCa.

References

1. Department of Health and Human Services. U.S. Cancer Statistics Working Group. United States cancer statistics: 1999–2014 incidence and mortality web-based report. Atlanta: U.S. Department of Health and Human Services; 2017.
2. Howlader NNA, Krapcho M, Miller D, Bishop K, Kosary CL, Yu M, Ruhl J, Tatalovich Z, Mariotto A, Lewis DR, Chen HS, Feuer EJ, Cronin KA. SEER cancer statistics review, 1975–2014. Bethesda, MD: National Cancer Institute; 2017.
3. Punnen S, Cooperberg MR. The epidemiology of high-risk prostate cancer. Curr Opin Urol. 2013;23(4):331–6.
4. Sanda MG, Dunn RL, Michalski J, Sandler HM, Northouse L, Hembroff L, et al. Quality of life and satisfaction with outcome among prostate-cancer survivors. N Engl J Med. 2008;358(12):1250–61.
5. Resnick MJ, Koyama T, Fan KH, Albertsen PC, Goodman M, Hamilton AS, et al. Long-term functional outcomes after treatment for localized prostate cancer. N Engl J Med. 2013;368(5):436–45.
6. Chaussy CG, Thuroff S. High-intensity focused ultrasound for the treatment of prostate cancer: a review. J Endourol. 2017;31(S1):S30–s7.
7. Thuroff S, Chaussy C. Evolution and outcomes of 3 MHz high intensity focused ultrasound therapy for localized prostate cancer during 15 years. J Urol. 2013;190(2):702–10.
8. Crouzet S, Chapelon JY, Rouviere O, Mege-Lechevallier F, Colombel M, Tonoli-Catez H, et al. Whole-gland ablation of localized prostate cancer with high-intensity focused ultrasound: oncologic outcomes and morbidity in 1002 patients. Eur Urol. 2014;65(5):907–14.
9. Ahmed HU. The index lesion and the origin of prostate cancer. N Engl J Med. 2009;361(17):1704–6.
10. Liu W, Laitinen S, Khan S, Vihinen M, Kowalski J, Yu G, et al. Copy number analysis indicates monoclonal origin of lethal metastatic prostate cancer. Nat Med. 2009;15(5):559–65.
11. Rischmann P, Gelet A, Riche B, Villers A, Pasticier G, Bondil P, et al. Focal high intensity focused ultrasound of unilateral localized prostate cancer: a prospective multicentric Hemiablation study of 111 patients. Eur Urol. 2017;71(2):267–73.
12. Feijoo ER, Sivaraman A, Barret E, Sanchez-Salas R, Galiano M, Rozet F, et al. Focal high-intensity focused ultrasound targeted hemiablation for unilateral prostate cancer: a prospective evaluation of oncologic and functional outcomes. Eur Urol. 2016;69(2):214–20.
13. Sanda MG, Crispino T, Freedland S, Greene K, Klotz LH, Makarov DV, Nelson JB, Reston J, Rodrigues G, Sandler HM, Taplin ME, Cadeddu JA. Clinically Localized Prostate Cancer: AUA/ASTRO/SUO Guideline. 2017.
14. NCCN Guidelines Version 2. 2017. Prostate Cancer Updates.
15. Passoni NM, Polascik TJ. How to select the right patients for focal therapy of prostate cancer? Curr Opin Urol. 2014;24(3):203–8.

16. Fulgham PF, Rukstalis DB, Turkbey IB, Rubenstein JN, Taneja S, Carroll PR, et al. AUA policy statement on the use of multiparametric magnetic resonance imaging in the Diagnosis, Staging and Management of Prostate Cancer. J Urol. 2017;198(4):832–8.

17. Ahmed HU, El-Shater Bosaily A, Brown LC, Gabe R, Kaplan R, Parmar MK, et al. Diagnostic accuracy of multi-parametric MRI and TRUS biopsy in prostate cancer (PROMIS): a paired validating confirmatory study. Lancet. 2017;389(10071):815–22.

18. Futterer JJ, Briganti A, De Visschere P, Emberton M, Giannarini G, Kirkham A, et al. Can clinically significant prostate cancer be detected with multiparametric magnetic resonance imaging? A systematic review of the literature. Eur Urol. 2015;68(6):1045–53.

19. Moldovan PC, Van den Broeck T, Sylvester R, Marconi L, Bellmunt J, van den Bergh RCN, et al. What is the negative predictive value of multiparametric magnetic resonance imaging in excluding prostate cancer at biopsy? A systematic review and meta-analysis from the European Association of Urology prostate cancer guidelines panel. Eur Urol. 2017;72(2):250–66.

20. Nassiri N, Chang E, Lieu P, Priester AM, Margolis DJA, Huang J, et al. Focal therapy eligibility determined by MRI/US fusion biopsy. J Urol. 2018;199(2):453–8.

21. Siddiqui MM, Rais-Bahrami S, Turkbey B, George AK, Rothwax J, Shakir N, et al. Comparison of MR/ultrasound fusion-guided biopsy with ultrasound-guided biopsy for the diagnosis of prostate cancer. JAMA. 2015;313(4):390–7.

22. Muller BG, Futterer JJ, Gupta RT, Katz A, Kirkham A, Kurhanewicz J, et al. The role of magnetic resonance imaging (MRI) in focal therapy for prostate cancer: recommendations from a consensus panel. BJU Int. 2014;113(2):218–27.

23. Jarow JP, Ahmed HU, Choyke PL, Taneja SS, Scardino PT. Partial gland ablation for prostate cancer: report of a Food and Drug Administration, American Urological Association, and Society of Urologic Oncology Public Workshop. Urology. 2016;88:8–13.

24. Muller BG, van den Bos W, Brausi M, Cornud F, Gontero P, Kirkham A, et al. Role of multiparametric magnetic resonance imaging (MRI) in focal therapy for prostate cancer: a Delphi consensus project. BJU Int. 2014;114(5):698–707.

25. Simmons LAM, Kanthabalan A, Arya M, Briggs T, Barratt D, Charman SC, et al. The PICTURE study: diagnostic accuracy of multiparametric MRI in men requiring a repeat prostate biopsy. Br J Cancer. 2017;116(9):1159–65.

26. Hovels AM, Heesakkers RA, Adang EM, Jager GJ, Strum S, Hoogeveen YL, et al. The diagnostic accuracy of CT and MRI in the staging of pelvic lymph nodes in patients with prostate cancer: a meta-analysis. Clin Radiol. 2008;63(4):387–95.

27. Wibmer AG, Burger IA, Sala E, Hricak H, Weber WA, Vargas HA. Molecular imaging of prostate cancer. Radiographics. 2016;36(1):142–59.

28. Postema AW, De Reijke TM, Ukimura O, Van den Bos W, Azzouzi AR, Barret E, et al. Standardization of definitions in focal therapy of prostate cancer: report from a Delphi consensus project. World J Urol. 2016;34(10):1373–82.

29. Le Nobin J, Rosenkrantz AB, Villers A, Orczyk C, Deng FM, Melamed J, et al. Image guided focal therapy for magnetic resonance imaging visible prostate cancer: defining a 3-dimensional treatment margin based on magnetic resonance imaging histology co-registration analysis. J Urol. 2015;194(2):364–70.

30. Schouten MG, van der Leest M, Pokorny M, Hoogenboom M, Barentsz JO, Thompson LC, et al. Why and where do we miss significant prostate cancer with multi-parametric magnetic resonance imaging followed by magnetic resonance-guided and transrectal ultrasound-guided biopsy in biopsy-naive men? Eur Urol. 2017;71(6):896–903.

31. Chaussy C, Thuroff S. The status of high-intensity focused ultrasound in the treatment of localized prostate cancer and the impact of a combined resection. Curr Urol Rep. 2003;4(3):248–52.

32. Vallancien G, Prapotnich D, Cathelineau X, Baumert H, Rozet F. Transrectal focused ultrasound combined with transurethral resection of the prostate for the treatment of localized prostate cancer: feasibility study. J Urol. 2004;171(6 Pt 1):2265–7.

Chapter 12
Radical Prostatectomy in the Metastatic Setting

Matteo Soligo, Vidit Sharma, and R. Jeffrey Karnes

Clinical Case Scenario: 62-year-old man who has multiple suspicious pelvic lymph nodes who desires aggressive therapy.

Is there a role for radical prostatectomy (RP) in the metastatic setting? For cN1 disease per NCCN guidelines, the suggested treatment is androgen deprivation therapy (ADT) ± radiation therapy (RT). However, the addition of RT to this treatment was not based on strong evidence. Nonetheless, it raises the question as to whether treatment to the primary treatment should be considered for metastatic disease, including cN1. A prototypical patient is presented to address the role of cytoreductive surgery for prostate cancer with clinical lymphadenopathy.

In this chapter, current evidence is provided regarding the putative advantages of cytoreductive RP, an intervention that has started to gain acceptance in the management of cN0/pN1—occult nodal metastatic disease—based on accumulating data over the last few decades that describe a survival advantage over systemic therapy alone. Even if several questions remain unanswered—such as the extent of nodal involvement and surgical dissection, the timing for ADT, and the incorporation of other systemic therapy and/or RT with ADT postoperatively—it does seem that patients with cN1 disease may benefit from a multimodal treatment approach. However, ideal patient selection remains uncertain for cytoreductive surgery, and further improvements are needed in detection of nodal disease.

M. Soligo, M.D. · V. Sharma, M.D. · R. Jeffrey Karnes, M.D., F.A.C.S. (✉)
Department of Urology, Mayo Clinic, Rochester, MN, USA
e-mail: soligo.matteo@mayo.edu; sharma.vidit@mayo.edu; karnes.r@mayo.edu

© Springer International Publishing AG, part of Springer Nature 2018   169
S. S. Chang, M. S. Cookson (eds.), *Prostate Cancer*,
https://doi.org/10.1007/978-3-319-78646-9_12

Case Description

Mr. S, a healthy 62-year-old gentleman, presents for evaluation and discussion regarding his first prostate biopsy, which he received for a cT3 exam and an initial PSA of 17.5 ng/dL. Biopsy revealed high-volume Gleason 4 + 3 = 7 in multiple cores with perineural invasion and extraprostatic extension. A staging multiparametric MRI (mpMRI) was performed and is partially depicted in Figs. 12.1 and 12.2. On the mpMRI, there are multifocal and diffuse PI-RADS 5 lesions with concomitant extracapsular extension and bilateral neurovascular bundle and right seminal vesicle invasion (not shown) in addition to pelvic lymphadenopathy. No distant metastases, either in the form of non-regional nodes, bone lesions, or visceral metastases, were visualized on his remaining staging scans.

In light of this clinical stage (cN1), according to the NCCN guidelines on prostate cancer, Mr. S is eligible for either:

- External beam radiation therapy (RT) + long-term androgen deprivation therapy (ADT)
- Long-term ADT alone

Fig. 12.1 Depiction of a deep right and left abnormal lymph nodes in the pelvis

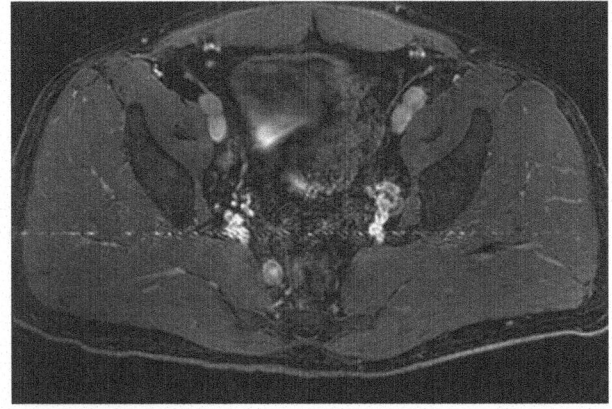

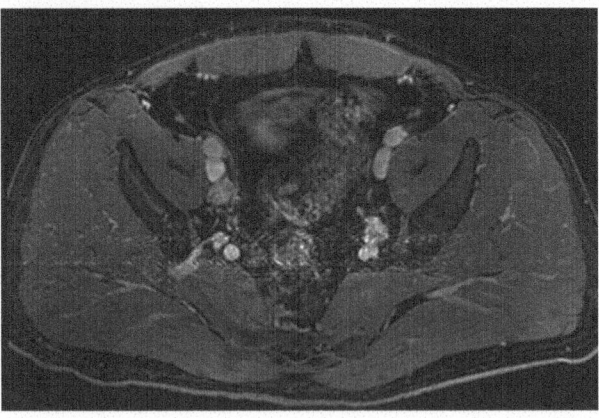

Fig. 12.2 Another suspicious right external iliac node

Mr. S learns the pros and cons of these two conventional therapeutic options that are recommended on relatively sparse data. Radical prostatectomy is not included in such guidelines statements, and there is poor quality retrospective evidence comparing RP to RT head-to-head in the cN1 setting. Mr. S explains that despite this guideline he wants to be as aggressive as possible and explore a multimodal approach.

Screening

PSA screening is a controversial topic often debated in the medical community. A Cochrane Review concluded that screening is associated with an increased number of prostate cancer (PCa) diagnoses but without a significant improvement in cancer-specific (CSS) nor overall survival (OS) [1]. On the other hand, the 2015 update to the European Randomized Study of Screening for Prostate Cancer (ERSPC) showed a 21% reduction in relative mortality at 13 years in the screened group. Importantly, the mortality reduction was not significant until 11 years of follow-up, highlighting the truly long-term outlook and life expectancy necessary to realize a screening benefit. One prostate cancer death was averted for 781 men screened and for 27 prostate cancers diagnosed [2]. Therein lies the dilemma of screening: balancing the harms of overdiagnosing [3] many clinically indolent cancers with the harms of missing a few aggressive cancers. However, the overdiagnosis side of the dilemma tended to receive more coverage in the lay press and academic circles outside of urology. Critics of PSA-based screening cited trends in overtreatment and loss in quality of life adjusted life years [4], leading the US Preventive Services Task Force (USPSTF) in 2008 (for men above the age of 75) and in 2012 (for all ages) to discourage routine PSA-based screening [5, 6].

The pendulum thus moved in the opposite direction as PSA screening declined and later-stage cancer became more frequent [7, 8]. In fact, the incidence of distant disease increased by ~1.4% per year from 2008 to 2013 in 50–74-year-old men [9]. This stage shift to more advanced disease makes the discussion of the role of RP in the management of cN1 more pertinent. The USPSTF continues to reevaluate its positions and has recently changed the screening recommendation to a grade C and emphasizes informed shared decisionmaking; it remains to be seen if the pendulum will swing back.

Diagnosis

The diagnosis of cN1 disease is relevant to this topic because several different imaging modalities exist detect to evaluate lymph nodes, each with varying sensitivity and specificity. Thus, the true burden of cN1 in question depends on the imaging modality used and has implications for comparing disease burden between patients and across series in the literature.

MRI

Multiparametric prostate (mp) MRI is gaining wider acceptance as a tool in the diagnosis and staging of prostate cancer [10]. More recently, MRI-targeted TRUS biopsy [11] has been associated with higher detection rates of clinically significant PCa compared to systematic biopsy(s) [12–15], while reducing the detection of clinically insignificant PCa [16, 17]. The last update to the Prostate Imaging Reporting and Data System (PI-RADS v2) [18] has also improved the accuracy of mpMRI. Further research is needed to merge MRI findings with clinical [19] data, such as PSA density [20], serum isoform [−2] proPSA [21], and prostate health index(*phi*) [22]. The PROMIS [17] (in the biopsy-naive setting) and PICTURE [23] (in the repeat biopsy setting) studies support the use of mpMRI, and the ongoing prospective non-randomized PROKOMB study is also expected to confirm the utility of mpMRI in initial staging/diagnosis [24]. Poor agreement among radiologists is another barrier to the dispersion of this modality [25, 26].

But there is still room to improve mpMRI's performance characteristics for extracapsular extension, seminal vesicle invasion [27], and regional node staging. It remains to be seen whether wider adoption of 3T scanners, dispersion of dynamic contrast enhanced sequences [28], and spectroscopic imaging [29] will improve the accuracy of mpMRI in reliably diagnosing clinical lymphadenopathy [30, 31]. Advancements in diffusion-weighted assessment of lymphadenopathy may yield further improvements in MRI characterization of lymph nodes [32]

Computed Tomography

Computed tomography (CT) is more commonly used for preoperative staging than mpMRI, but with its ubiquity comes a reduced accuracy [30] particularly when it comes to tumor staging [31]. CT mainly relies on size, contour, enhancement, and internal architecture. There is still debate on defining radiographic lymphadenopathy for prostate cancer in terms of dimension cutoffs. Often evolution of the lymphadenopathy (either in response to ADT or over time) is used to confirm indeterminate findings.

PET

Positron emission tomography (PET) has been employed in initial staging, either localized or advanced disease. ^{11}C-choline, ^{18}F-choline, and ^{11}C-acetate have been the first tracers to be widely employed related to their ability to detect increased lipid metabolism [33]. Sensitivity and specificity estimates for primary tumor staging vary widely, with detection rates ranging from 11 to 100% according to a meta-analysis [33]. There are also studies exploring the utility for choline PET-CT in the assessment of lymph node invasion [34]. While the specificity is 90%, the main limitation to its sensitivity (around 40%) is due to the tendency to miss pathologic lymph nodes below 0.4 cm [35]. Up to 45% metastatic nodes are smaller than this size.

^{68}Gallium-labeled prostate-specific membrane antigen PET/CT (^{67}Ga-PSMA PET/CT) may have more potential for nodal staging. A recent review found this tracer to be more sensitive (61%) and just as specific as 11C-choline and 18F-choline (97%) in delineating nodal metastasis [36]. Two ongoing trials—^{68}Ga-PSMA PET: Evaluation of Gallium-HBED-CC-PSMA Imaging in Prostate Cancer patients (PSMA PET), NCT02611882, and ^{68}Ga-PSMA PET/MRI in Finding Tumors in Patients with Intermediate or High-Risk Prostate Cancer Undergoing Surgery, NCT02678351—are expected to give further clarification. It also remains to be seen if these imaging modalities can improve clinical nomograms predicting positive nodes on lymphadenectomy, such as the Briganti nomogram [37].

Evaluation

Once the diagnosis of cN1 is suspected (likely based on conventional CT or MRI), the evaluation that ensues usually varies considerably from the standard prostate cancer work-up. Risk of distant metastatic disease has to be considered. Thus, in addition to pelvic imaging, abdominal imaging and a bone scan are necessary. It has also been our preference to evaluate the chest, usually with a chest CT.

The value of nodal biopsy has not been clearly defined in this setting. We rarely advocate for nodal biopsies, and usually they are performed in situations where it would dramatically change the treatment preference of the patient. But when they are performed, it is vital to perform them under CT guidance with an experienced interventional radiology team given the proximity to vasculature.

It is important to note the number and location of the pelvic lymph nodes. It has been our experience that positive nodes out of the true pelvis (such as the low para-aortic and para-caval) represent higher-risk disease. Furthermore, it is important to understand that grade is still an independent prognostic factor in the setting. In other words, Gleason 7 (4 + 3) with lymphadenopathy is a different player than Gleason 9 (4 + 5) with lymphadenopathy. Furthermore, treatment may not be appropriate for every cN1 PCa patient. A multicenter study reminds us that non-PCa-related mortality is relevant in older patients with comorbidities [38]. Appreciating the whole clinical picture is thus vital to judge cancer mortality for an individual and inform the treatment discussions to follow.

Therapeutic Management

Radical Prostatectomy

Evidence Supporting Radical Prostatectomy in N+ Disease

Radical prostatectomy is not included in guidelines for the management of cN1 or other metastatic disease states of PCa. This is largely based on "historic" belief that nodal invasion by PCa is emblematic of widespread systemic disease precluding local treatment. But much of the reported data refute this notion. Several potential biologic mechanisms support that RP should be explored in the cN1 and metastatic setting: cytoreduction, the removal of the primary source of future cellular dissemination, and the restoration of antitumor immunity [39]. An interesting translational study by Tzelepi et al. found persistent viable PCa foci with active metastatic pathways within the prostate in spite of a 1-year course of ADT and three cycles of taxane-based and many with undetectable PSAs [40]. Further, Gannon et al. introduced the concept that the alterations in the nodal microenvironment with immunosuppressive cytokines and tumor growth-promoting factors might enhance further metastasis [41]. Another study expounded on these findings and characterized T-cell suppression in this nodal microenvironment [42].

Surgical series investigating the role of RP plus hormonal therapy vs. hormonal therapy alone in the setting of pN1 date back to the late 1960s [43, 44]. Likely due to the poor quality of CTs at that time, many of these men would most likely now be cN1 or cM1 today. Engel et al. used a population-based German registry and found an OS and CSS benefit with RP on multivariable analysis [43]. Ghavamian et al. performed a matched-controlled analysis and reported RP + adjuvant orchiectomy had a significant 10-year OS and CSS survival advantage over pelvic lymphadenectomy and orchiectomy only [44]. Using this same patient study cohort, Bhindi et al. found that RP and orchiectomy were superior to orchiectomy alone at 20 years with a HR of 0.48 in favor of RP and orchiectomy for OS [45]. The 10-year OS and CSS for RP + ADT have been quite consistent and among different studies/institutions (around 55%–75% and 60%–85%, respectively) and superior than ADT alone (28% and 40.5–46%) [46]. This is also consistent with randomized trial of adjuvant or deferred ADT in pN1 after RP (ECOG 3886 [47]), in which adjuvant ADT had a 65% 10-year OS.

Perhaps the most striking evidence in favor of radical prostatectomy in the setting of lymphadenopathy comes from a series in which prostatectomies would often be aborted in the presence of pathologically positive nodes. Steuber et al. [48] compared 50 patients who had RP aborted due to positive nodes intraoperatively to 108 patients who had their RP completed. Both groups received adjuvant ADT postoperatively. At 10 years, cancer-specific survival was 46% in the aborted RP group compared to 76% in the completed RP group. In essence, patients who had RP aborted had excisional lymph node biopsies and did much worse than the completion RP cohort. Both groups were clearly operative candidates and thus presumably had similar comorbidities. Although it is unknown in regard to the clinical nodal burden, this data demonstrates the benefit of RP in the setting of lymphadenopathy.

More recently, reviews have summarized retrospective series to support the role of RP in pN1 and M1 patients [49, 50]. RP with EPLND included in multimodal regimens provided a better survival benefit in advanced disease over a single modality [51, 52]. A recent study based on 2967 patients from the National Cancer Database supported the belief that local therapy (either RP or RT) is superior to ADT in improving OS and CSS in cN1 disease; however, it failed to find a statistically significant difference between RT + ADT and RP + ADT [53].

Extent of Lymphadenectomy During Radical Prostatectomy

In the presence of clinical lymphadenopathy, there are few studies examining the effect of PLND extent and oncologic outcomes. Without clinical lymphadenopathy, MRI findings have not added to the reliability of detecting clinically occult lymph nodes and have not improved on clinical nomogram's prediction of lymph nodal invasion [54, 55]. For instance, the updated Briganti nomogram has an 87.6% AUC in predicting the probability of lymph node invasion (LNI). Despite some encouraging findings of a sentinel lymph node-based nomogram [56, 57], a recent consensus statement did not support omitting extended PLND based on sentinel node assessment in intermediate- and high-risk prostate cancer [58]. Thus, for high-risk patients, including cN1 patients, we advocate a meticulous, visually complete removal of the external iliac, obturator, internal iliac, presacral, and common iliac lymph node packets up to the boundary of the ureteric crossing. This usually yields a minimum of 20 nodes, but it is critical to visually complete the dissection as opposed to obtaining a minimal nodal count. In practice, we will often incorporate more proximal common iliac and para-caval and para-aortic nodes. It is important to note that it is rare for prostate cancer to have positive retroperitoneal nodes without positive pelvic nodes, although we have noticed a few of these cases. It has been our practice to send nodes for intraoperative frozen section to confirm that the clinically positive nodes have indeed been removed. We also want to know if there are nodes outside of the true pelvis (such as common iliac or low retroperitoneal) that are positive to help determine recurrence risk. While it is controversial, we do believe that removing more nodes within the nodal drainage of the prostate is associated with improved oncologic outcomes. But it is important to interpret retrospective series that report such claims with caution as it is difficult to adjust for the Will-Rogers phenomenon completely [59].

Prognosis of pN1 Patients After Radical Prostatectomy

The heterogeneous prognosis of pN1 patients after radical prostatectomy suggests that a subset of patients may not have micrometastatic disease at the time of surgery and may experience prolonged disease-free survival after radical prostatectomy. Moschini et al. [60] found that one-third of RP patients with pN1 disease managed with adjuvant hormonal therapy will experience a clinical recurrence by 15 years postoperatively, and 50% of these still recur in the pelvis, arguing against "universal" systemic disease. Many studies support that increased number of positive nodes portends a worse prognosis [61–63]. In the largest and longest study on pN1 disease from a single center (n = 1011 pN1 patients with a median follow-up of 17.6 years), Moschini et al. identified the following favorable prognostic features: less than two positive nodes, pathological Gleason score 6 or 7, negative surgical margins, and receipt of adjuvant radiotherapy [64]. Carlsson et al. [65] reported that the extranodal extension, the volume of the node with a pathological cancer focus, and the volume of the metastatic focus (linear extent) within the node had a negligible impact on survival outcome. On the other hand, other prognostic factors should be taken in account, such as surgical Gleason score [66], positive surgical margins, extracapsular extension, and seminal vesicle invasion [67].

Evidence for Radical Prostatectomy in M1 Disease

There is a growing body of evidence supporting radical prostatectomy in the M1 setting, and this supports a benefit for RP in the cN1 setting. Culp et al. queried SEER for 8185 M1a-c patients undergoing either brachytherapy, RP, or no local therapy and found that RP was associated with the best survival [68]. Moschini et al. [69] demonstrated that perioperative RP outcomes were similar to RP [70, 71] in the nonmetastatic setting: positive surgical margin rate of 26%, lymphocele rate of 6.5%, anastomosis leak rate of 3.2%, wound infection rate of 6.5%, and 3month continence of 77%. A multi-institutional series by Sooriakumaran et al. [72] also supported the feasibility cytoreductive prostatectomy.

Primary Radiation Therapy

Radiation therapy (RT) is a currently recommended treatment for cN1 patients, usually with concomitant ADT. In fact, this is our treatment of choice for patients who are not operative candidates but still have a life expectancy of 10 years. In the primary setting, RT plus ADT has been shown to be associated with improved survival via population-based cancer databases [53, 73, 74]. In clinically node-negative patients, there is evidence supporting RT and ADT over ADT alone in PCa with higher-risk features [75, 76]. Currently, most guidelines would agree that 2–3 years of ADT is recommended with radiation therapy. The benefit of whole pelvic nodal irradiation in the presence of cN1 disease is not yet established. However, conceptually, we do agree that the nodal field should be included in the presence of clinical lymphadenopathy.

Hypofractionation, in which higher doses per session are administered, has not been found to have an increase in side effects on surrounding tissues [77]. This has also been employed in the postoperative setting for pN1 for fossa and nodal radiation with acceptable toxicity [78].

Postoperative Radiotherapy

If a radical prostatectomy is performed with clinical lymphadenopathy, considerations for postoperative radiotherapy are often part of the clinical course. Adjuvant RT has been associated with improved survival in pN1 by large retrospective series [79, 80]. In our own series, we find that adjuvant RT confers a cancer-specific survival advantage to no adjuvant RT in patients with pN1 disease [64]. In another multi-institutional cohort, Touijer et al. [81] found that adjuvant ADT + RT was associated with improved overall survival for pN1 patients. A recent systematic review found that adjuvant RT is associated with improved survival for pN1 patients [82]. Accurate patient selection is still a matter of debate: a retrospective study by Abdollah et al. on 1107 pN1 patients treated with RP + ADT found that adjuvant RT was helpful for patients with up to four positive lymph nodes depending on primary tumor characteristic [63]. A large percentage of pN1 patients will also have seminal vesicle invasion, and Moschini et al. [83] also found that patients with SVI + pN1 may be more likely to benefit from adjuvant RT.

Timing of RT is another controversial issue: is adjuvant better than early salvage? A retrospective study on 773 pN1 patients out of the Martini Klinik [84] who underwent adjuvant RT had a lower metastasis rate than salvage RT patients (8.2% vs. 17.5% at 4 years). However, in the same series, early salvage radiotherapy (given at PSA < 0.50) was found to be better than late salvage. Since early salvage RT was not compared to adjuvant RT, the jury is still out in terms of timing.

In practice, we prefer to administer radiotherapy once the patient's incontinence has come down to one pad per day or less. Usually this occurs by the 3-month mark postoperatively, and we also have the results of the first PSA check. Thus, the line between early salvage and adjuvant RT is often blurred. Patients with one positive node at the time of surgery may simply be observed if the primary tumor is not pT3 and no positive margins. On the other hand, patients with three or more positive nodes usually get multimodal treatment with adjuvant RT (often with whole pelvic) and ADT. Patients with two positive nodes are managed with a combination of these approaches.

Systemic Therapies

Androgen Deprivation Therapy

ADT has been the cornerstone for the treatment of metastatic PCa. Rarely do we employ preoperative ADT in cN1 unless there is a concern for resectability of the primary tumor or if the patient is unable to schedule surgery for several months. In the postoperative setting for pN1, the ECOG 3886 trial (Messing trial) [47] suggested that adjuvant ADT immediately postoperatively was associated with improved survival. Another trial, EORTC 30846 [85], found that when the prostate was left in situ, immediate vs. delayed ADT was similar. In our practice, patients with three or more nodes usually receive adjuvant ADT for the long term with consideration of hormone therapy holidays. The decision for patients with one or two positive nodes is more individualized and also depends on the use of adjuvant radiotherapy, in which case ADT is used to complement the radiotherapy.

Novel Androgen Agents: Abiraterone

Novel agents acting on the androgen pathway are of significant interest in the prostate cancer community. Recently, trials have found that one of these agents, abiraterone, may be useful in the hormone-sensitive state. The STAMPEDE group followed 1917 patients with mainly untreated prostate cancer (95%) with either high-risk node-negative (28%), node-positive (20%), or metastatic (52%) disease randomized to abiraterone + prednisolone + standard of care (ADT ± RT) against standard of care [86]. In the nonmetastatic subset, abiraterone was associated with significantly improved progression-free survival than standard of care (~90% vs. 70% at 3 years) but not overall survival. The trial did not stratify the nonmetastatic population into cN0 and cN1 in its forest plots, but presumably the progression-free survival advantage is maintained for the cN1M0 patient. The results of another recent trial, LATITUDE [87], supported that abiraterone had a ~15% 3-year overall survival benefit relative to ADT alone for men with newly diagnosed metastatic hormone-sensitive prostate cancer with 2/3 of the following features: Gleason ≥8, ≥ bone metastases or visceral metastasis. However, this trial cannot be directly applied to our patient in the cN1M0 setting.

Chemotherapy

The role of docetaxel for newly diagnosed cN1 disease (without distant metastasis) is controversial. There are three trials in the metastatic disease space: GETUG-AFU15 [88], CHAARTED [89], and STAMPEDE [90] trials, all investigated combined ADT + docetaxel. However, for all of these trials, it is not clear how many cN1M0 patients fit in the "low-volume disease" groups.

The original GETUG-AFU 15[89] was the first phase III study to compare ADT + docetaxel vs. ADT alone. The trial did find an improved biochemical progression-free survival for the chemotherapy group but did not find an overall survival difference for either high-volume or low-volume disease, even at extended follow-up [91].

CHAARTED [89] was the first randomized trial to show a survival improvement for ADT + docetaxel over ADT alone in a cohort of 790 men with newly diagnosed hormone-sensitive PCa, most of them (72.8%) naive to previous local treatment of PCa. It is unclear how many cN1M0 patients were in the low-volume group, for which our index patient would fit closer to. The hazard ratio for overall survival for ADT + docetaxel was 0.61 ($p < 0.001$) for the overall cohort and 0.60 ($p < 0.001$) for the high-volume group (defined as visceral involvement and/or ≥ 4 bone metastasis, of which at least 1 outside the spine or pelvis) and 0.61 ($p = 0.11$) for the low-volume group. There were 513 patients in the high-volume group and 277 patients in the low-volume group. The presence of the same hazard ratio favoring ADT + docetaxel in the high-volume and low-volume subsets but a p-value of 0.11 opens that possibility for the trial being underpowered in the low-volume subset. But with the data we have at hand, it is unlikely that our cN1M0 patient would stand to benefit from ADT + docetaxel on the basis of the CHAARTED trial.

STAMPEDE trial [90] largely confirmed CHAARTED findings supporting the use of docetaxel in the metastatic setting. However, there were only 171 cN1M0 patients in the control arm and 86 in the docetaxel arm. Looking at the subset of M0 patients as a whole (some of whom were N0 and some N1), docetaxel did not have a survival benefit (HR 95% confidence interval, 0.62–1.47). However, STAMPEDE included locally advanced N0M0 patients (if there were two of the following: T3/4, Gleason 8–10, PSA > 40 ng/mL), and investigators did not do a subset survival analysis for cN1M0 patients. Instead they grouped the cN0M0 and cN1M0 groups together, and thus we cannot confidently apply the trial to our index patient. In practice, we tend to extrapolate the findings from the M0 subset (of whom about half had cN0 and half had cN1) and do not advocate for docetaxel therapy in this setting.

Concluding Remarks

Going back to our index patient: 62-year-old male with "multiple suspicious pelvic nodes" desiring aggressive treatment. The guidelines would provide a simple choice: ADT alone vs. radiotherapy + ADT, with most healthy men likely choosing the latter. However, in our experience, well-selected cN+ patients can be offered radical prostatectomy. In fact, our group recently found that among 302 men found to be pN1 at radical prostatectomy, cN1 patients had similar 15-year cancer-specific mortality compared to cN0 patients (30% vs. 31%, $p = 0.6$) [92]. Multiple studies as outlined before have demonstrated a benefit of RP over ADT alone in the N1M0 setting. Thus, we would not hesitate to offer a patient radical prostatectomy with an extended PLND (including removal of the low retroperitoneal nodes in some cases) if he is healthy and interested in an aggressive approach. Preoperative counseling would be extensive, and we would emphasize that there is a high chance of a multimodal approach. Postoperative ADT will often be advocated if the number of positive nodes is three or more or if he has pT3b and one or two nodes positive. Postoperative radiotherapy to the fossa and whole pelvis will also often be delivered (again depending on the patient's risk) when the patient has regained continence and is usually given in conjunction with ADT. Lastly, we would risk stratify his disease postoperatively and have him understand his overall prognosis based on our models detailed in this chapter. We would discuss that if the patient is toward the higher-risk spectrum, then the inclusion of abiraterone with ADT may provide a progression-free survival benefit, and insurance approval for pN1M0 indication is awaited. We, however, would not advocate for postoperative docetaxel therapy Undoubtedly, randomized clinical trials would improve our current knowledge as it pertains to multimodal approaches to lymph node -only metastatic disease especially when confined within the pelvis.

References

1. Hayes JH, Barry MJ. Screening for prostate cancer with the prostate-specific antigen test: a review of current evidence. JAMA. 2014;311:1143–9.
2. Schröder FH, et al. Screening and prostate cancer mortality: results of the European randomised study of screening for prostate cancer (ERSPC) at 13 years of follow-up. Lancet. 2014;384:2027–35.
3. Draisma G, et al. Lead time and overdiagnosis in prostate-specific antigen screening: importance of methods and context. J Natl Cancer Inst. 2009;101:374–83.
4. Wilt TJ, Dahm P. PSA screening for prostate cancer: why saying no is a high-value health care choice. J Natl Compr Cancer Netw. 2015;13:1566–74.
5. US Preventive Services Task Force. Screening for prostate cancer: US. preventive services task force recommendation statement. Ann Intern Med. 2008;149:185–91.
6. Moyer VA, US Preventive Services Task Force. Screening for prostate cancer: U.S. preventive services task force recommendation statement. Ann Intern Med. 2012;157:120–34.
7. Jemal A, SA F, Ma J, al e. Prostate cancer incidence and psa testing patterns in relation to uspstf screening recommendations. JAMA. 2015;314:2054–61.
8. Li J, Berkowitz Z, Hall IJ. Decrease in prostate cancer testing following the US preventive services task force (USPSTF) recommendations. J Am Board Fam Med. 2015;28:491–3.
9. Fleshner K, Carlsson SV, Roobol MJ. The effect of the USPSTF PSA screening recommendation on prostate cancer incidence patterns in the USA. Nat Rev Urol. 2017;14:26–37.
10. Yoo S, Kim JK, Jeong IG. Multiparametric magnetic resonance imaging for prostate cancer: a review and update for urologists. Korean J Urol. 2015;56:487–97.
11. Wegelin O, et al. Comparing three different techniques for magnetic resonance imaging-targeted prostate biopsies: a systematic review of in-bore versus magnetic resonance imaging-transrectal ultrasound fusion versus cognitive registration. Is there a preferred technique? Eur Urol. 2017;71:517–31.
12. van Hove A, et al. Comparison of image-guided targeted biopsies versus systematic randomized biopsies in the detection of prostate cancer: a systematic literature review of well-designed studies. World J Urol. 2014;32:847–58.
13. Siddiqui MM, et al. Comparison of MR/ultrasound fusion–guided biopsy with ultrasound-guided biopsy for the diagnosis of prostate cancer. JAMA. 2015;313:390–7.
14. Valerio M, et al. Detection of clinically significant prostate cancer using magnetic resonance imaging-ultrasound fusion targeted biopsy: a systematic review. Eur Urol. 2015;68:8–19.
15. Schoots IG, et al. Magnetic resonance imaging-targeted biopsy may enhance the diagnostic accuracy of significant prostate cancer detection compared to standard Transrectal ultrasound-guided biopsy: a systematic review and meta-analysis. Eur Urol. 2015;68:438–50.
16. Meng X, et al. Relationship between prebiopsy multiparametric magnetic resonance imaging (MRI), biopsy indication, and MRI-ultrasound fusion-targeted prostate biopsy outcomes. Eur Urol. 2016;69:512–7.
17. Ahmed HU, et al. Diagnostic accuracy of multi-parametric MRI and TRUS biopsy in prostate cancer (PROMIS): a paired validating confirmatory study. Lancet. 2017;389:815–22.

18. Weinreb JC, et al. PI-RADS prostate imaging—reporting and data system: 2015, version 2. Eur Urol. 2016;69:16–40.
19. Radtke JP, et al. Combined clinical parameters and multiparametric magnetic resonance imaging for advanced risk modeling of prostate cancer—patient-tailored risk stratification can reduce unnecessary biopsies. Eur Urol. 2017;72(6):888–96. https://doi.org/10.1016/j.eururo.2017.03.039.
20. Venderink W, et al. Results of targeted biopsy in men with magnetic resonance imaging lesions classified equivocal, likely or highly likely to be clinically significant prostate cancer. Eur Urol. 2017. https://doi.org/10.1016/j.eururo.2017.02.021.
21. Furuya K, et al. Measurement of serum isoform [−2]proPSA derivatives shows superior accuracy to magnetic resonance imaging in the diagnosis of prostate cancer in patients with a total prostate-specific antigen level of 2–10 ng/ml. Scand J Urol. 2017;51:251–7.
22. Tosoian JJ, et al. Prostate health index density improves detection of clinically significant prostate cancer. BJU Int. 2017;120(6):793–8. https://doi.org/10.1111/bju.13762.
23. Simmons LAM, et al. The PICTURE study: diagnostic accuracy of multiparametric MRI in men requiring a repeat prostate biopsy. Br J Cancer. 2017;116:1159–65.
24. Baur ADJ, et al. A prospective study investigating the impact of multiparametric MRI in biopsy-naïve patients with clinically suspected prostate cancer: the PROKOMB study. Contemp Clin Trials. 2017;56:46–51.
25. Muller BG, et al. Prostate cancer: interobserver agreement and accuracy with the revised prostate imaging reporting and data system at multiparametric MR imaging. Radiology. 2015;277:741–50.
26. Hansen NL, et al. Comparison of initial and tertiary centre second opinion reads of multiparametric magnetic resonance imaging of the prostate prior to repeat biopsy. Eur Radiol. 2017;27:2259–66.
27. Hamoen EHJ, de Rooij M, Witjes JA, Barentsz JO, Rovers MM. Eur Urol. 2015;67:1112–21.
28. Radtke JP, Teber D, Hohenfellner M, Hadaschik BA. The current and future role of magnetic resonance imaging in prostate cancer detection and management. Transl Androl Urol. 2015;4(3):326–41.
29. Cabarrus MC, Westphalen AC. Multiparametric magnetic resonance imaging of the prostate—a basic tutorial. Transl Androl Urol. 2017;6:376–86.
30. Kiss B, Thoeny HC, Studer UE. Current status of lymph node imaging in bladder and prostate cancer. Urology. 2016;96:1–7.
31. Hövels AM, et al. The diagnostic accuracy of CT and MRI in the staging of pelvic lymph nodes in patients with prostate cancer: a meta-analysis. Clin Radiol. 2008;63:387–95.
32. Thoeny HC, Froehlich JM, Triantafyllou M, Bains LJ, Vermathen P. Metastases in normal-sized pelvic lymph nodes: detection with diffusion-weighted MR imaging. Radiology. 2014;273:125–35.
33. Evangelista L, et al. New clinical indications for 18 F/11 C-choline, new tracers for positron emission tomography and a promising hybrid device for prostate cancer staging: a systematic review of the literature. Eur Urol. 2016;70:161–75.
34. Brogsitter C, Zöphel K, Kotzerke J. 18F-Choline, 11C-choline and 11C-acetate PET/CT: comparative analysis for imaging prostate cancer patients. Eur J Nucl Med Mol Imaging. 2013;40:18–27.
35. Evangelista L, Guttilla A, Zattoni F, Muzzio PC, Zattoni F. Utility of choline positron emission tomography/computed tomography for lymph node involvement identification in intermediate- to high-risk prostate cancer: a systematic literature review and meta-analysis. Eur Urol. 2013;63:1040–8.
36. von Eyben FE, Picchio M, von Eyben R, Rhee H, Bauman G. 68Ga-labeled prostate-specific membrane antigen ligand positron emission tomography/computed tomography for prostate cancer: a systematic review and meta-analysis. Eur Urol Focus. 2016. https://doi.org/10.1016/j.euf.2016.11.002.
37. Gandaglia G, et al. Development and internal validation of a novel model to identify the candidates for extended pelvic lymph node dissection in prostate cancer. Eur Urol. 2017;72:632–40.

38. Briganti A, et al. Impact of age and comorbidities on long-term survival of patients with high-risk prostate cancer treated with radical prostatectomy: a multi-institutional competing-risks analysis. Eur Urol. 2013;63:693–701.
39. da Costa WH, Guimarães GC. Radical prostatectomy in metastatic prostate cancer: is there enough evidence? I opinion: yes. Int Brazilian J Urol. 2016;42:876–9.
40. Tzelepi V, et al. Persistent, biologically meaningful prostate cancer after 1 year of androgen ablation and docetaxel treatment. J Clin Oncol. 2011;29:2574–81.
41. Gannon PO, et al. Presence of prostate cancer metastasis correlates with lower lymph node reactivity. Prostate. 2006;66:1710–20.
42. Sharma V, Dong H, Kwon E, Karnes RJ. Positive pelvic lymph nodes in prostate cancer harbor immune suppressor cells to impair tumor-reactive T cells. Eur Urol Focus. 2016. https://doi.org/10.1016/j.euf.2016.09.003.
43. Engel J, et al. Platinum priority—prostate cancer survival benefit of radical prostatectomy in lymph node—positive patients with prostate cancer. Eur Urol. 2010;57:754–61.
44. Ghavamian R, Bergstralh EJ, Blute MJ, Slezak J, Zincket H. Radical retropubic prostatectomy plus orchiectomy versus orchiectomy alone for pTxN+ prostate cancer: a matched comparison. J Urol. 1999;161:1223–8.
45. Bhindi B, et al. Impact of radical prostatectomy on long-term oncologic outcomes in a matched cohort of men with pathological node positive prostate cancer managed by castration. J Urol. 2017;198:86–91.
46. Gakis G, et al. The role of radical prostatectomy and lymph node dissection in lymph node—positive prostate cancer: a systematic review of the literature. Eur Urol. 2014;66:191–9.
47. Messing EM, et al. Immediate versus deferred androgen deprivation treatment in patients with node-positive prostate cancer after radical prostatectomy and pelvic lymphadenectomy. Lancet Oncol. 2006;7:472–9.
48. Steuber T, et al. Radical prostatectomy improves progression-free and cancer-specific survival in men with lymph node positive prostate cancer in the prostate-specific antigen era: a confirmatory study. BJU Int. 2011;107:1755–61.
49. Veeratterapillay R, Goonewardene SS, Barclay J, Persad R, Bach C. Radical prostatectomy for locally advanced and metastatic prostate cancer. Ann R Coll Surg Engl. 2017;99:259–64.
50. Moschini M, Soria F, Briganti A, Shariat SF. The impact of local treatment of the primary tumor site in node positive and metastatic prostate cancer patients. Prostate Cancer Prostatic Dis. 2017;20:7–11.
51. Fahmy O, Khairul-Asri MG, Hadi SHSM, Gakis G, Stenzl A. The role of radical prostatectomy and radiotherapy in treatment of locally advanced prostate cancer: a systematic review and meta-analysis. Urol Int. 2017;99:249–56.
52. Fossati N, et al. The benefits and harms of different extents of lymph node dissection during radical prostatectomy for prostate cancer: a systematic review. Eur Urol. 2017;72:84–109.
53. Seisen T, et al. Efficacy of local treatment in prostate cancer patients with clinically pelvic lymph node-positive disease at initial diagnosis. Eur Urol. 2017. https://doi.org/10.1016/j.eururo.2017.08.011.
54. Cagiannos I, et al. A preoperative nomogram identifying decreased risk of positive pelvic lymph nodes in patients with prostate cancer. J Urol. 2003;170:1798–803.
55. Briganti A, et al. Updated nomogram predicting lymph node invasion in patients with prostate cancer undergoing extended pelvic lymph node dissection: the essential importance of percentage of positive cores. Eur Urol. 2012;61:480–7.
56. Winter A, et al. Updated Nomogram incorporating percentage of positive cores to predict probability of lymph node invasion in prostate cancer patients undergoing sentinel lymph node dissection. J Cancer. 2017;8:2692–8.
57. Grivas N, et al. Validation and head-to-head comparison of three nomograms predicting probability of lymph node invasion of prostate cancer in patients undergoing extended and/or sentinel lymph node dissection. Eur J Nucl Med Mol Imaging. 2017;44(13):2213–26. https://doi.org/10.1007/s00259-017-3788-z.

58. van der Poel HG, et al. Sentinel node biopsy for prostate cancer: report from a consensus panel meeting. BJU Int. 2017;120:204–11.
59. Abdollah F, et al. More extensive pelvic lymph node dissection improves survival in patients with node-positive prostate cancer. Eur Urol. 2015;67:212–9.
60. Moschini M, et al. Natural history of clinical recurrence patterns of lymph node-positive prostate cancer after radical prostatectomy. Eur Urol. 2017;69:135–42.
61. Seay TM, Blute ML, Zincke H. Long-term outcome in patients with pTxN+ adenocarcinoma of prostate treated with radical prostatectomy and early androgen ablation. J Urol. 1998;159:357–64.
62. Schiavina R, et al. Differing risk of cancer death among patients with lymph node metastasis after radical prostatectomy and pelvic lymph node dissection: identification of risk categories according to number of positive nodes and Gleason score. BJU Int. 2013;111:1237–44.
63. Abdollah F, et al. Impact of adjuvant radiotherapy on survival of patients with node-positive prostate cancer. J Clin Oncol. 2014;32:3939–47.
64. Moschini M, et al. Risk stratification of pN+ prostate cancer after radical prostatectomy from a large single institutional series with long-term followup. J Urol. 2016;195:1773–8.
65. Carlsson SV, et al. Pathological features of lymph node metastasis for predicting biochemical recurrence after radical prostatectomy for prostate cancer. J Urol. 2013;189:1314–9.
66. Touijer KA, Mazzola CR, Sjoberg DD, Scardino PT, Eastham JA. Long-term outcomes of patients with lymph node metastasis treated with radical prostatectomy without adjuvant androgen-deprivation therapy. Eur Urol. 2014;65:20–5.
67. Nguyen DP, et al. Updated postoperative nomogram incorporating the number of positive lymph nodes to predict disease recurrence following radical prostatectomy. Prostate Cancer Prostatic Dis. 2017;20:105–9.
68. Culp SH, Schellhammer PF, Williams MB. Might men diagnosed with metastatic prostate cancer benefit from definitive treatment of the primary tumor? A SEER-Based Study. Eur Urol. 2014;65:1058–66.
69. Moschini M, Morlacco A, Kwon E, Rangel LJ, Karnes RJ. Treatment of M1a/M1b prostate cancer with or without radical prostatectomy at diagnosis. Prostate Cancer Prostatic Dis. 2017;20:117–21.
70. Tewari A, et al. Positive surgical margin and perioperative complication rates of primary surgical treatments for prostate cancer: a systematic review and meta-analysis comparing retropubic, laparoscopic, and robotic prostatectomy. Eur Urol. 2012;62:1–15.
71. Ficarra V, et al. Systematic review and meta-analysis of studies reporting urinary continence recovery after robot-assisted radical prostatectomy. Eur Urol. 2012;62:405–17.
72. Sooriakumaran P, et al. A multi-institutional analysis of perioperative outcomes in 106 men who underwent radical prostatectomy for distant metastatic prostate cancer at presentation. Eur Urol. 2016;69:788–94.
73. Lin CC, Gray PJ, Jemal A, Efstathiou JA. Androgen deprivation with or without radiation therapy for clinically node-positive prostate cancer. J Natl Cancer Inst. 2015;107:djv119.
74. Rusthoven CG, et al. The impact of definitive local therapy for lymph node-positive prostate cancer: a population-based study. Int J Radiat Oncol. 2014;88:1064–73.
75. Fosså SD, et al. Ten- and 15-yr prostate cancer-specific mortality in patients with nonmetastatic locally advanced or aggressive intermediate prostate cancer, randomized to lifelong endocrine treatment alone or combined with radiotherapy: final results of the Scandinavian. Eur Urol. 2016;70:684–91.
76. Mason MD, et al. Final report of the intergroup randomized study of combined androgen-deprivation therapy plus radiotherapy versus androgen-deprivation therapy alone in locally advanced prostate cancer. J Clin Oncol. 2015;33(19):2143–50.
77. Koontz BF, Bossi A, Cozzarini C, Wiegel T, D'Amico A. A systematic review of hypofractionation for primary management of prostate cancer. Eur Urol. 2015;68:683–91.
78. Van Hemelryk A, et al. The outcome for patients with pathologic node-positive prostate cancer treated with intensity modulated radiation therapy and androgen deprivation therapy: a case-matched analysis of pN1 and pN0 patients. Int J Radiat Oncol. 2016;96:323–32.

79. Briganti A, et al. Combination of adjuvant hormonal and radiation therapy significantly prolongs survival of patients with pT2–4 pN + prostate cancer: results of a matched analysis. Eur Urol. 2011;59:832–40.
80. Abdollah F, et al. Selecting the optimal candidate for adjuvant radiotherapy after radical prostatectomy for prostate cancer: a long-term survival analysis. Eur Urol. 2013;63:998–1008.
81. Touijer KA, et al. Survival outcomes of men with lymph node-positive prostate cancer after radical prostatectomy: a comparative analysis of different postoperative management strategies. Eur Urol. 2017. https://doi.org/10.1016/j.eururo.2017.09.027.
82. Mano R, Eastham J, Yossepowitch O. The very-high-risk prostate cancer: a contemporary update. Prostate Cancer Prostatic Dis. 2016;19:340–8.
83. Moschini M, et al. Long-term utility of adjuvant hormonal and radiation therapy for patients with seminal vesicle invasion at radical prostatectomy. BJU Int. 2017;120:69–75.
84. Tilki D, et al. Adjuvant radiation therapy is associated with better oncological outcome compared with salvage radiation therapy in patients with pN1 prostate cancer treated with radical prostatectomy. BJU Int. 2017;119:717–23.
85. Schröder FH, et al. Early versus delayed endocrine treatment of T2-T3 pN1-3 M0 prostate cancer without local treatment of the primary tumour: final results of European Organisation for the Research and Treatment of Cancer protocol 30846 after 13 years of follow-up (a randomised controlled trial). Eur Urol. 2009;55:14–22.
86. James ND, et al. Abiraterone for prostate cancer not previously treated with hormone therapy. N Engl J Med. 2017;377:338–51.
87. Fizazi K, et al. Abiraterone plus prednisone in metastatic, castration-sensitive prostate cancer. N Engl J Med. 2017;377:352–60.
88. Gravis G, et al. Androgen-deprivation therapy alone or with docetaxel in non-castrate metastatic prostate cancer (GETUG-AFU 15): a randomised, open-label, phase 3 trial. Lancet Oncol. 2013;14:149–58.
89. Sweeney CJ, et al. Chemohormonal therapy in metastatic hormone-sensitive prostate cancer. N Engl J Med. 2015;373:737–46.
90. James ND, et al. Addition of docetaxel, zoledronic acid, or both to first-line long-term hormone therapy in prostate cancer (STAMPEDE): survival results from an adaptive, multiarm, multistage, platform randomised controlled trial. Lancet. 2016;387:1163–77.
91. Gravis G, et al. Androgen deprivation therapy (ADT) plus docetaxel versus ADT alone in metastatic non castrate prostate cancer: impact of metastatic burden and long-term survival analysis of the randomized phase 3 GETUG-AFU15 trial. Eur Urol. 2016;70:256–62.
92. Moschini M, et al. Outcomes for patients with clinical lymphadenopathy treated with radical prostatectomy. Eur Urol. 2016;69:193–6.

Chapter 13
Resection of Metastatic Cancer in Castration-Resistant Patients

Justin R. Gregg, Chad Reichard, and John Davis

Clinical Case Scenario: 57-year-old man who underwent prostatectomy and lymph node dissection who develops CRPC, but only persistent active site is a large left pelvic lymph node.

What We Know and Do Not Know About Options and Outcomes

The scenario facing the above patient involves the management of castration-resistant prostate cancer (CRPC) in the setting of prior prostatectomy with lymphadenectomy with likely disease recurrence in a pelvic lymph node. Treating this patient is both nuanced and complicated given the rapidly evolving management of advanced prostate cancer and paucity of data guiding salvage lymphadenectomy in the castration-resistant setting. Options for treatment include multiple modalities, including systemic therapies (such as chemotherapy) that have proven efficacy in the metastatic CRPC setting [1], and localized treatment such as radiation or surgery. This chapter aims to outline the issues and reasoning behind various treatment options for patients with CRPC and local disease recurrence and specifically updates evidence related to salvage lymphadenectomy in this setting.

J. R. Gregg, M.D. · C. Reichard, M.D. · J. Davis, M.D. (✉)
Department of Urology, The University of Texas MD
Anderson Cancer Center, Houston, TX, USA
e-mail: JRGregg@mdanderson.org; CAReichard@mdanderson.org

© Springer International Publishing AG, part of Springer Nature 2018   185
S. S. Chang, M. S. Cookson (eds.), *Prostate Cancer*,
https://doi.org/10.1007/978-3-319-78646-9_13

How Does This Scenario Occur? What Does It Mean for The Patient?

Large series with extended follow-up demonstrate that up to 35% of men who undergo radical prostatectomy for localized adenocarcinoma have a biochemical recurrence at some point during follow-up [2, 3]. While biochemical recurrence precedes systemic disease in men who have previously been treated for prostate cancer, not all men with biochemical recurrence are destined to have metastases. A large retrospective cohort of men who had prostatectomy did not undergo neoadjuvant or adjuvant treatment and had biochemical recurrence revealed that 11.7% developed systemic recurrence and 5.8% died from prostate cancer (while 17.1% died from other causes). Multivariate analysis revealed that patient age, Gleason score, tumor stage, and PSA doubling time were associated with systemic progression and death [4], results that were similar to prior analyses [5]. Notably, this study included a large proportion of patients who did not harbor aggressive prostate cancer given that those requiring systemic treatment before or after treatment were excluded and over 50% of patients had a pathologic Gleason score ≤ 6 (grade group 1). Among men at increased risk of disease recurrence who were excluded from this study, level 1 evidence exists that adjuvant radiation therapy lowers the risk of disease recurrence and may improve overall survival. However, even with adjuvant radiation, approximately 23% of patients will have a biochemical recurrence within 5 years [6].

The mainstay of treatment for men with progressive and metastatic prostate cancer is androgen deprivation therapy via medical or surgical castration [7]. CRPC is therefore defined as prostate cancer that continues to progress (often as measured by the PSA) despite castration levels of testosterone [1]. While castration resistance is not curable, one-third of men who have CRPC develop bone metastases within 2 years, and the median metastasis-free survival was shown to be 30 months in a randomized study [8]. These results likely indicate that, even among men with CRPC, there is heterogeneity in terms of disease aggression and many have an extended time period before the development of detectable metastasis. Given that oligometastasis may represent a kind of intermediate tumor with limited metastatic capabilities [9], CRPC may have a theoretical window during which aggressive local disease control may offer a survival benefit, even in the presence of nodal disease.

Diagnostic Considerations

However, given the proven efficacy of systemic therapies in the presence of distant metastatic disease [1, 10], effort should be made to exclude extrapelvic disease prior to consideration of localized treatment for recurrent nodal CRPC, as its presence may change clinical management. Traditionally, axial imaging with or without 11C positron emission tomography (PET) was used in conjunction with bone scans to delineate both local and distant metastases; however, emerging diagnostic tests, such as sodium fluoride F18 [11] and ^{68}Ga-labeled prostate-specific membrane antigen PET bone scans [12], may offer improved sensitivity and specificity, even at low PSA values [13]. It is important to caution, though, that most ongoing trials investigating the efficacy of oligometastatic prostate cancer treatment rely on conventional imaging, and invasive treatment decisions made based on scans with improved diagnostic abilities are currently considered experimental [14].

What About Systemic Therapy Only?

Provided diagnostic work-up does not reveal systemic metastases, consideration should first be given to the use of systemic treatment modalities with androgen deprivation therapy. The reasoning for this is twofold. First, there is increasing evidence that systemic therapies used in metastatic CRPC treatment are effective at prolonging survival when moved up earlier in the treatment algorithm [1]. Second, systemic therapy does not preclude concurrent localized therapy, especially given that CRPC patients will already be on systemic antiandrogens by definition (this contrasts with management of men with castration-sensitive disease, where localized treatment may provide oncologic benefit while potentially delaying or obviating the need for androgen deprivation [15]). In terms of systemic agents that may be effective in this population, recent studies have shown that the antiandrogen enzalutamide [16] and the androgen synthesis inhibitor abiraterone (with prednisone) [17] improve overall survival when given before docetaxel chemotherapy, which was previously the standard of care for metastatic CRPC [18]. While these trials were completed in men with castration-sensitive prostate cancer and did not include men with isolated local disease (e.g., pelvic lymphadenopathy), prespecified subgroup analyses did examine factors that may be reflective of disease bulk. Subgroups based on baseline PSA, lactate dehydrogenase, alkaline phosphatase levels [16, 17], the presence of bony metastases [17], and the presence of visceral metastases [16] did not show survival differences, though multivariable analyses did show some association with overall survival (highlighting a potentially prognostic value).

Further evidence may be gleaned from a recent randomized trial of abiraterone and prednisone with androgen deprivation therapy vs. androgen deprivation therapy alone in patients with castration-sensitive disease [19]. While full subgroup analyses are not available, the study included 38 patients with recurrent disease after prior treatment who were randomized to ADT alone and 60 similar patients randomized to combination therapy. The use of combination therapy in these groups was not associated with overall survival (HR 0.94 [0.35–2.52]) though was associated with improved failure-free survival (HR 0.32 [0.16–0.65]). Notably, of the 38 patients randomized to ADT alone, 26 (68.4%) had metastatic disease at trial entry, compared to 35 (58.3%) combination therapy patients. The fact that 15–16% of patients across the study who had metastases were nodal, only, likely indicates that these groups were at a higher risk of recurrence than patients with isolated local disease recurrence, potentially diminishing the benefit of abiraterone in these lower-risk patients. While future subgroup analyses may provide further insight regarding combination therapy response in patients with oligometastatic nodal disease, this trial was not powered for this type of endpoint and does not offer substantive data to suggest that abiraterone use in this population is indicated outside of clinical trials. Similarly, other second-generation antiandrogen drugs have not been evaluated in the non-metastatic CRPC setting, though trials are ongoing [20]. Other systemic treatments that are considered in metastatic CRPC include docetaxel chemotherapy, the immune therapy sipuleucel-T and radium-223 dichloride [18, 20]. Unfortunately, these, too, have not been evaluated in the setting of low-volume locally recurrent disease and are therefore not included in this review.

What About Surgical Resection?

Regardless of whether systemic treatment is given to men with CRPC and pelvic lymph node recurrences, the option remains to provide localized therapy. Importantly, data is limited regarding the performance and outcomes of a salvage lymph node dissection in this setting. At the authors' institution, some evidence may be gleaned from patients in whom prostatectomy was performed in the setting of CRPC (unpublished). Among a very small group of men who underwent prostatectomy and extended lymph node dissection for CRPC, 1/9 (11%) with clinically node-positive disease did not have disease on final pathology, indicating that node positivity may have a high-sensitivity disease presence in this (albeit small) population. In terms of CRPC in the setting of clinically positive pelvic lymphadenopathy, a total of three retrospective reviews have investigated the use of salvage node dissection in men with CRPC, all of which highlight the potential limitations of this approach while simultaneously offering evidence regarding the safety of its use (Table 13.1).

In a 2012 study by Busch et al., six patients received salvage lymph node dissection after primary treatment and subsequent development of castration resistance. Three patients had previously undergone prostatectomy, two radiotherapy, and one androgen deprivation with lymph node dissection. Preoperatively, the mean PSA was 37.6 ng/dL. Template usage varied, with three undergoing a unilateral template, two with a bilateral template, and one a bilateral extended dissection. No operative-related complications were observed. Postoperatively, patients did see an average PSA decline of 39.3%, and PSA velocity dropped by 11.2 months. However, 4/6 (67%) patients developed bone metastases at a median time period of 23.5 months [21].

Zattoni et al. published a large cohort of men who underwent salvage LN dissection following prostatectomy in 2016 [22]. While many of the patients had androgen-sensitive disease, 22 patients (18.8%) had CRPC. All patients had radiologic evidence of disease based on 11C PET/CT imaging, and all underwent an extended

Table 13.1 Summary of studies evaluating salvage pelvic lymphadenectomy in patients with CPRC

Study	Total # patients	Total # CRPC	PSA response	Other outcomes	Complications
Busch [21]	6	6	Average decline of 39.3% and PSA velocity dropped to 11.2 months	4/6 (67%) developed postoperative bone metastases at a median of 23.5 months	None
Zattoni [22]	117	22	All but one patient had a postoperative "decline"	No pre- or postoperative variables associated with biochemical recurrence in CRPC patients	23/1117 (19.7%). four (3.4%) grade IIIa, two (1.7% grade IIIb
Osmonov [23]	54	43	31 patients (68.9%) had a postoperative decline to a mean of PSA 4.4, representing a 34.3% decrease	Ten patients (22.2%) eventually developed bone metastases, seven died. 24 patients (53.3%) with CRPC responded to androgen deprivation following nod dissection	7/54 (15.6%). All grade IIIb

template that included tissue removal in the external and internal iliac, obturator fossa, and presacral and common iliac vessels up to the aortic bifurcation. Overall, 23 of 117 (19.7%) patients had a complication: four (3.4%) were Clavien-Dindo Grade IIIa, two (1.7%) were IIIb, and one (0.8%) was IVa. In terms of postoperative outcomes, subgroup analyses of the CRPC group were not performed, though the authors did note that all patients in the cohort had a postoperative PSA decline except for one. In fact, over 80% of patients had a PSA decline to <0.2 ng/dL; however, the majority of patients received androgen deprivation therapy postoperatively (as would be expected for the CRPC group). Notably, 5-year biochemical recurrence-free survival was 31% for the entire cohort, though it must be assumed that this rate was higher in the CRPC group given the presence of more aggressive disease. Among 19 pre- and postoperative variables examined for association with biochemical recurrence after salvage lymph node dissection in the subgroup of patients with CRPC, none were associated with recurrence.

Finally, a 2016 study by Osmonov et al. detailed results of salvage lymphadenectomy performed in a cohort of 54 patients, 43 (80%) of whom had CRPC. All patients underwent a preoperative 11C PET/CT, and indications for surgery included lymph node-positive disease or biochemical recurrence with PSA over 0.5 ng/dL. Operative templates were similar to those used in the study by Zattoni et al. Complications were observed in seven patients (15.6%), all of which were Clavien IIIb: two bleeding, two with ureteral stricture, one rectovesical fistula (the cohort included ten patients who underwent salvage prostatectomy following radiotherapy, as well), and two lymphoceles. Of the entire cohort, 31 patients (68.9%) had a postoperative decline in PSA. Mean preoperative PSA was 6.7, with a mean postoperative nadir of 4.4 (34.3% decline). During an average follow-up of 42.7 months, biochemical recurrence-free survival for the entire cohort was 30% (though the rate was unclear for the CRPC subgroup). Ten patients (22.2%) developed bone metastases during follow-up, and seven patients died. Interestingly, 24 patients with preoperative CRPC (53.3%) responded to ADT initially following node dissection [23].

Based on these data, salvage lymph node dissection following prostatectomy and subsequent lymph node recurrence can be safely performed with an acceptably low (but not zero) complication rate. While patient numbers are small and total follow-up is not ideal, there is strong evidence that most patients benefit from an initial decline in PSA. Due to a lack of comparator groups, conclusions cannot be drawn regarding the effect of salvage node dissection in CRPC patients on time to biochemical recurrence and development of metastases. However, it is intriguing that the study reported by Osmonov et al. offered evidence of renewed response to androgen deprivation therapy in the CRPC group, theorized to be related to the removal of particularly aggressive prostate cancer cells present in removed lymph nodes [23]. These data provide evidence for the continued investigation of localized treatment in the setting of CRPC through clinical trials.

Surgical Resection: Technical Considerations

Given the limited available evidence on efficacy and numerous different clinical scenarios, it is useful for surgeons from tertiary centers with experience to comment on operating in these conditions.

- In the index case described, the patient has an enlarged pelvic lymph node. This will mean that the surgeon will likely have a visible target to extirpate and have reasonable confidence when the target lymph node is removed along with the desired templates listed. Figure 13.1 shows a sequence of removing grossly enlarged nodes in a patient on ADT and early CRPC.
- In other circumstances, the surgeon may be dealing with a lymph node(s) that is not enlarged but identified by functional imaging such as PET. These cases may prove challenging as there may not be a clear target node seen at surgery. Rather, the imaging has to be translated into an accurate template of resection, and measurement of success may not be available until final pathology, follow-up imaging, and/or biochemical response. PET images need to be shown in fused format both coronal and sagittal.
- Given that the efficacy of resection is unclear, it is reasonable to proceed with the "attitude" that these endeavors must be kept low morbidity. When target lymph nodes occur along extended pelvic lymph node fields commonly resected during radical prostatectomy or cystectomy, then success should be achievable. Figure 13.2 shows a sequence of dissections involving the common iliacs above the ureter, presacral, and periaortic to the IMA. However, when lymph nodes are involving "out-of-bounds" locations such as the mesorectum, then caution is warranted as injury to the gastrointestinal tract is probably not worth the risk. Furthermore, lymph nodes high up in the retroperitoneum require a more elabo-

rate surgical approach and likely represent a different disease biology and may not be indicated at this time.

- Previous lymph node surgery makes a difference. In our experience, a unilateral extended pelvic lymph node dissection takes on average 20 min as a pri-

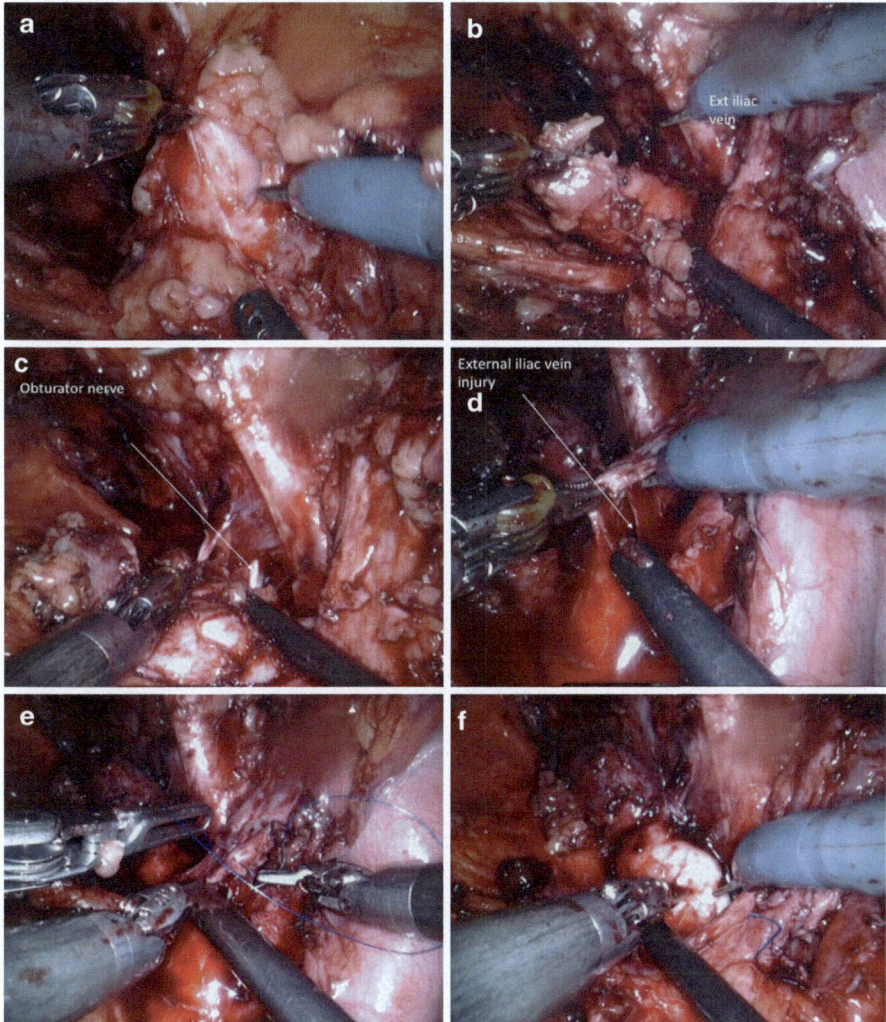

Fig. 13.1 Grossly involved lymph nodes on the right after 6 months ADT. (**a**) Pale/firm nodal mass encountered immediately upon dissecting into the right external iliac chain. (**b**) The obturator space nodes could be disconnected from the node of Cloquet. (**c**) The obturator nerve is visible distally but nodal mass creating a challenge to expose and protect. (**d**) Dissecting between the external iliac artery and vein proximally created a vein injury. (**e**) The vein injury is small, easy to repair with 3-0 PDS figure of eight. (**f**) Gross nodal involvement continues under the external iliac vein, requiring dissection from multiple angles. (**g**) Dissection lateral to the external iliac artery. (**h**) Dissection along the common iliac artery to the ureteral crossing. (**i**) Dissection between the external iliac artery and vein. (**j**) Dissection continues down the hypogastric chain

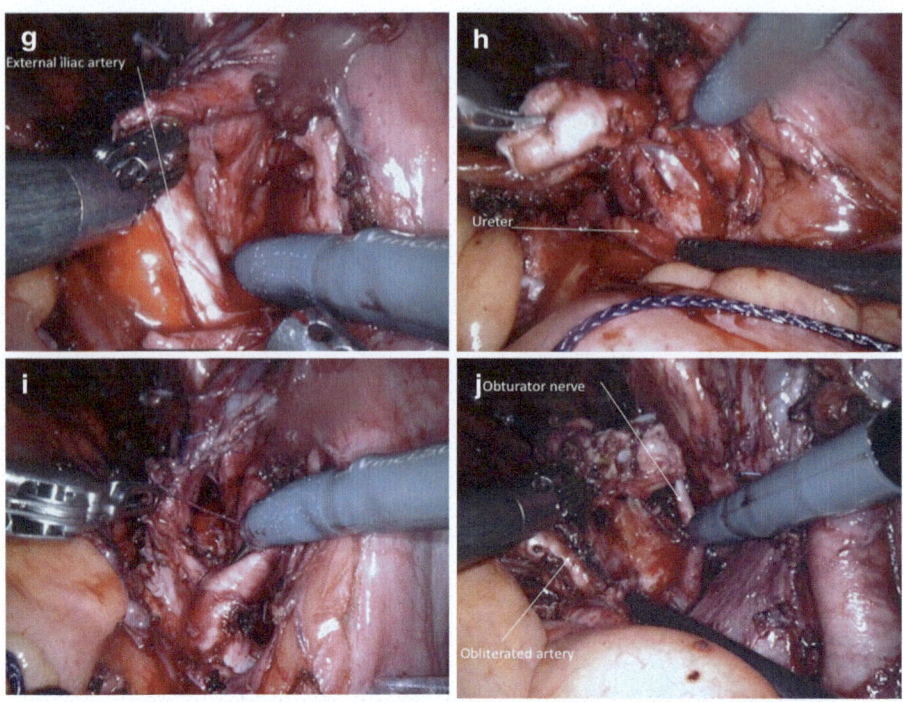

Fig. 13.1 (continued)

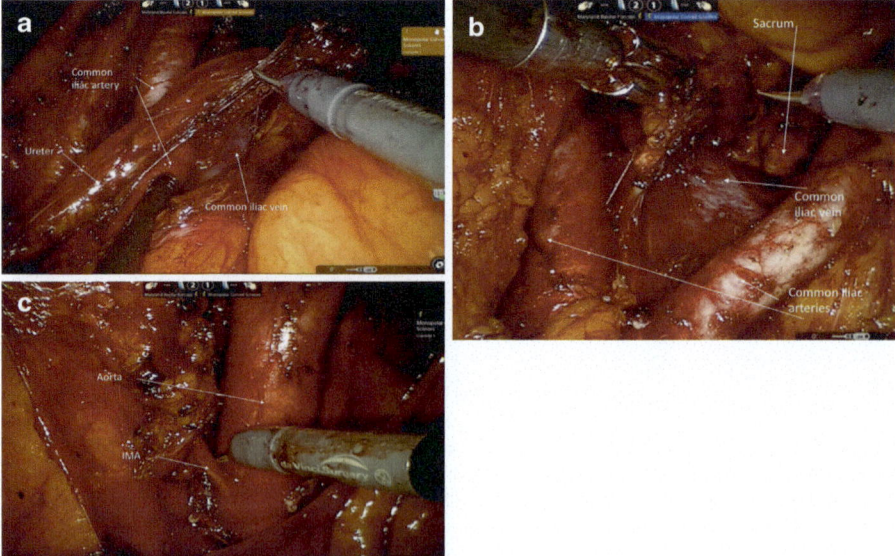

Fig. 13.2 Higher PLND dissections for salvage/very high-risk indications. (**a**) Left common iliac dissection above/below ureter. (**b**) Presacral dissection. (**c**) Aortic dissection to the inferior mesenteric artery

mary procedure, 30–40 min as a salvage/previously untouched procedure, and 90 or more minutes as a salvage/previous PLND procedure. The latter is not uncommon, as many surgeons still believe in a "standard" PLND template for some circumstances, and having to dissect that template into an extended dissection requires greater effort to free up the vessels and obturator nerve without injury.

- In general, prior robot, laparoscopic, or even open radical prostatectomy as a single procedure (i.e., no nodes) will not create much surgical challenge in access to nodes.

What About the Radiation Options?

Further evidence regarding the possible efficacy of salvage local treatment for radiographically detected lymph in men with CRPC can be found in the limited literature related to salvage radiation therapy. Two studies that examined the effects of radiation therapy completed for oligometastatic disease included CRPC patients, though both involved radiation of metastases (rather than local lymphatic disease). The first by Tabata et al. [24] involved selective radiation of all metastatic bone lesions in men with fewer than six metastases. The study was a retrospective review of 35 patients, seven of whom (20%) had CRPC. While PSA response is not detailed, radiation dosing had no effect on overall survival on multivariable analysis, which included CRPC as a covariate. A study by Ahmed et al. used similar inclusion criteria in reporting treatment outcomes of 17 patients, 11 of whom had CRPC, who received radiation therapy to five or fewer bone metastases [25]. Among all patients, PSA declined at the first post-radiotherapy visit with the exception of two patients who had immediate distant progression. When considering only patients with CRPC, at a median follow-up of 4.8 months, 6 men (55%) had an undetectable or continuously down-trending PSA. While clearly offering the possibility of a PSA decline, further studies are needed to both confirm this benefit and evaluate clinically relevant outcomes in men with CRPC and low-volume metastases who undergo targeted radiotherapy. Multiple ongoing trials are designed to evaluate these outcomes, including two studies that include only men with CRPC [20].

Summation

Given these data, the potential benefits of salvage local control of recurrent CRPC are promising, including the potential to limit disease bulk and slow the rate of progression, as evidenced by PSA declines following therapy. However, at this juncture, improvements in relevant outcomes such as biochemical progression and survival are purely theoretical. Further study in locally recurrent CRPC is warranted, making surgical intervention a potentially valuable option that may be used in the future as part of an evolving multidisciplinary approach to men with CRPC. The authors are hopeful that clinical trials focused on local disease control in men with castration-sensitive disease (NCT01751438, NCT02454543, and NCT02138721 on clinicaltrials.gov) will offer further insights regarding the benefits of local oligometastatic disease treatment and will lead to additional investigations in the CRPC population. Until that time, though promising, extirpative therapy focused on local recurrence in the setting of CRPC remains experimental and should be completed through approved protocols and explicit patient consent and would not be recommended for use in the patient introduced at the beginning of this chapter as a standard of care.

References

1. Cookson MS, Roth BJ, Dahm P, et al. Castration-resistant prostate cancer: AUA Guideline. J Urol. 2013;190:429–38.
2. Roehl KA, Han M, Ramos CG, et al. Cancer progression and survival rates following anatomical radical retropubic prostatectomy in 3,478 consecutive patients: long-term results. J Urol. 2004;172:910–4.
3. Han M, Partin AW, Pound CR, et al. Long-term biochemical disease-free and cancer-specific survival following anatomic radical retropubic prostatectomy. Urol Clin North Am. 2001;28:555–65.
4. Boorjian SA, Thompson RH, Tollefson MK, et al. Long-term risk of clinical progression after biochemical recurrence following radical prostatectomy: the impact of time from surgery to recurrence. Eur Urol. 2011;59:893–9.
5. Freedland SJ, Humphreys EB, Mangold LA, et al. Risk of prostate cancer-specific mortality following biochemical recurrence after radical prostatectomy. JAMA. 2005;294:433–9.
6. Daly T, Hickey BE, Lehman M, et al. Adjuvant radiotherapy following radical prostatectomy for prostate cancer. Cochrane Database Syst Rev. 2011:CD007234.
7. Loblaw DA, Virgo KS, Nam R, et al. Initial hormonal management of androgen-sensitive metastatic, recurrent, or progressive prostate cancer: 2007 update of an American Society of Clinical Oncology Practice Guideline. J Clin Oncol. 2007;25:1596–605.
8. Smith MR, Kabbinavar F, Saad F, et al. Natural history of rising serum prostate-specific antigen in men with castrate nonmetastatic prostate cancer. J Clin Oncol. 2005;23:2918–25.
9. Weichselbaum RR, Hellman S. Oligometastases revisited. Nat Rev Clin Oncol. 2011;8:378–82.
10. Cornford P, Bellmunt J, Bolla M, et al. EAU-ESTRO-SIOG guidelines on prostate cancer. Part II: treatment of relapsing, metastatic, and castration-resistant prostate cancer. Eur Urol. 2017;71:630–42.
11. Talbot JN, Paycha F, Balogova S. Diagnosis of bone metastasis: recent comparative studies of imaging modalities. Q J Nucl Med Mol Imaging. 2011;55:374–410.
12. Perera M, Papa N, Christidis D, et al. Sensitivity, specificity, and predictors of positive 68 Ga–prostate-specific membrane antigen positron emission tomography in advanced prostate cancer: a systematic review and meta-analysis. Eur Urol. 2016;70:926–37.
13. Bach-Gansmo T, Nanni C, Nieh PT, et al. Multisite experience of the safety, detection rate and diagnostic performance of Fluciclovine ((18)F) positron emission tomography/computerized tomography imaging in the staging of biochemically recurrent prostate cancer. J Urol. 2017;197:676–83.
14. Murphy DG, Sweeney CJ, Tombal B. "Gotta catch 'em all'", or do we? Pokemet approach to metastatic prostate cancer. Eur Urol. 2017;72:1–3.

15. Ploussard G, Almeras C, Briganti A, et al. Management of node only recurrence after primary local treatment for prostate cancer: a systematic review of the literature. J Urol. 2015;194:983–8.
16. Beer TM, Armstrong AJ, Rathkopf DE, et al. Enzalutamide in metastatic prostate cancer before chemotherapy. N Engl J Med. 2014;371:424–33.
17. Ryan CJ, Smith MR, de Bono JS, et al. Abiraterone in metastatic prostate cancer without previous chemotherapy. N Engl J Med. 2013;368:138–48.
18. Tannock IF, de Wit R, Berry WR, et al. Docetaxel plus prednisone or mitoxantrone plus prednisone for advanced prostate cancer. N Engl J Med. 2004;351:1502–12.
19. James ND, de Bono JS, Spears MR, et al. Abiraterone for prostate cancer not previously treated with hormone therapy. N Engl J Med. 2017;377:338–51.
20. Wei XX, Ko EC, Ryan CJ. Treatment strategies in low-volume metastatic castration-resistant prostate cancer. Curr Opin Urol. 2017;27(6):596–603.
21. Busch J, Hinz S, Kempkensteffen C, et al. Selective lymph node dissection for castration-resistant prostate cancer. Urol Int. 2012;88:441–6.
22. Zattoni F, Nehra A, Murphy CR, et al. Mid-term outcomes following salvage lymph node dissection for prostate cancer nodal recurrence status post-radical prostatectomy. Eur Urol Focus. 2016;2:522–31.
23. Osmonov DK, Aksenov AV, Trick D, et al. Cancer-specific and overall survival in patients with recurrent prostate cancer who underwent salvage extended pelvic lymph node dissection. BMC Urol. 2016;16:56.
24. Tabas I. Consequences of cellular cholesterol accumulation: basic concepts and physiological implications. J Clin Invest. 2002;110:905–11.
25. Ahmed KA, Barney BM, Davis BJ, et al. Stereotactic body radiation therapy in the treatment of oligometastatic prostate cancer. Front Oncologia. 2012;2:215.

Index

© Springer International Publishing AG, part of Springer Nature 2018
S. S. Chang, M. S. Cookson (eds.), *Prostate Cancer*,
https://doi.org/10.1007/978-3-319-78646-9

The manufacturer's authorised representative in the EU is Springer
Nature Customer Service Centre GmbH, Europaplatz 3, 69115 Heidelberg,
Germany. If you have any concerns regarding our products, please
contact ProductSafety@springernature.com

Printed and bound by CPI Group (UK) Ltd, Croydon, CR0 4YY

29/04/2026

02099451-0003